CHIMERA CONFLICT

A BOSTON BRAIN
IN A UYGHUR BODY

CHIMERA CONFLICT

A BOSTON BRAIN
IN A UYGHUR BODY

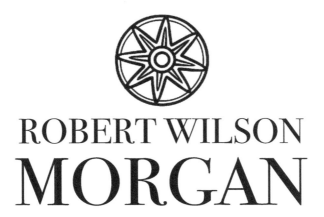

ROBERT WILSON
MORGAN

PROLOGUE

A chimera is an organism with more than one source of DNA. U.S. surgeons create about 40,000 human chimeras every year through successful organ transplants. Chinese surgeons do many more. In 2017, in China, Dr. Ren reported the first human head transplant after years of animal experimentation. There were mixed reactions in the scientific community. China has been severely criticized for its high transplant rate by using condemned prisoners as organ donors.

Although his team has not reported more head or brain transplants, it would seem plausible that they have continued to perfect head and brain transplants without publicity.

This novel is a fictional account of a severely injured American doctor, Roger Scully, who takes advantage of the Chinese expertise to have his brain transplanted into a prisoner's body. The ensuing chimera resumes his medical career in China as Dr. Wu Zicheng. He attempts to resuscitate his American career as Dr. Roger Scully, though not without several adventures and continuing problems over his identity.

CHAPTER 1

The constant hiss of a leaking pipe. A metal clang. Unfamiliar voices speaking in strange tongues. Then memories, with sound echoing through his brain. Bars of Mom's lullaby. Dad exhorting him to "skate harder." Riffs from his guitar. A familiar voice reading something. "What can you say about a twenty-five-year-old girl who died?"

Is that from Love Story?

Confusion.

Am I dreaming?

His body shook as someone moved his limbs. More sensations. This time from his skin. Rubbing, kneading, punching?

Why does someone keep turning me over?

He moved his right arm and hit a metal rail.

A hospital bed?

I can't think.

His eyes were shut, but his head was filled with lights.

It's like a 4th of July fireworks show in my head.

White lights, then colors, flashed from every angle, mixed with more memories. Mom's tongue-out smile while cuddling him. Dad holding him up on skates. Freckles on Joanne's face. The scene from the top of the ski run.

And oh, memories of falls. Into the pool at the Y, down the front stairs at home, the crashing end of his first bike ride, a spectacular wipeout on his skis. And now, the most terrifying free fall of all, like tumbling through space.

What's happening to me?

What's that smell?

An antiseptic tang.

Is that real or remembered?

The scent of chocolate chip cookies baking. Burgers on the barbecue. The sweet, floral aroma of a woman's perfume.

"Zicheng, wake up! Zicheng, wake up!"

Who is that man shouting? Who is Zicheng?

"Roger, wake up! Roger, wake up!"

Roger brightened on hearing his name. *They're calling me.* He opened his eyes and looked toward the voice but saw only a shadowy shape. *Is that a head? Is someone staring at me over the rails of my bed?* Through a blur, he saw a man in a white coat bending over him. Roger tried to speak, but only air came out. He was unable to make a sound.

"Zicheng, move your hands and feet," the man commanded.

Roger didn't know who Zicheng was, but the order was clear enough, and he tried to obey. He wasn't sure if he was moving his limbs or not. *Why am I in a hospital? And this isn't Denver General.*

"I am Dr. Li, and you are in Harbin, in China, in hospital," the man said. "You have had major surgery and have been asleep for a long time. You cannot speak right now, but I need to know if you can hear me. If you hear me, blink your eyes twice."

Roger blinked twice. With intense concentration and effort, he tried to speak, but no sound came out. *Oh shit, a tracheostomy. Why do they keep calling me Zicheng?*

For the next twenty minutes, Dr. Li gave various commands for movement—a voice coming through the sound of hissing water.

Roger's vision varied from quite clear to hopelessly muddled, with flashes of light at random times. *Let me sleep. Stop the torture.*

When he kept his eyes shut and refused to respond with blinks, Li said, "Okay, Zicheng, you can go back to sleep for a while, but you will wake up again, and you're going to get very much better. Tonight, we will plug your tracheostomy, so you will be able to speak again."

Darkness. Slipping under the surface to a sound sleep had never felt so good.

CHAPTER 2

Confusion continued for two days, but Roger became better oriented and aware of his surroundings. Why was this woman reading *Love Story* aloud? He could not understand why he found it difficult to speak, even with the tracheostomy closed. His tongue tangled when he tried to verbalize words from his thoughts; he did not recognize the voice when he spoke. He drank through a straw and ate some semi-liquid food; he tasted nothing. His ears continued hissing. Between visual flashes, Roger frowned at the Mandarin Good Luck plaque on the wall.

Everything he touched felt strange; had someone frozen his thick fingers with a local anesthetic? He moved his arms. They did not feel like his own. He felt as though his legs were detached.

Concentrating, he moved his right wrist into view. Squinting at the plastic wristband, he made out a series of Chinese characters and, in English, *Wu Zicheng*. No mention of Roger Scully.

He touched his forehead. *Was that a suture line?* He traced its ridge across the brow, skull top, and back of his neck. Brain surgery would explain his constant ringing headache. An attendant removed his catheter. Two nurses helped him stand briefly, but he could not walk. Roger felt as though he had no control over his body and legs. The nurses who insisted he stand to pee did not reply to his questions.

On Thursday, his first day fully awake, instead of hearing Dr. Li's shouted orders, he heard, "Hello, my sweet Zicheng. Did you think I would forget you? I've been coming every day to read to you while you slept in your coma." He looked up, saw a familiar face, and he felt pleasure but was not sure why. Her Asian face wore too-large glasses and a wide smile. In her medical student's jacket, she clutched a paperback novel. So she was the one who had been reading *Love Story*.

"Your operation was a big success," she said. "Your doctors asked me to come from Chengdu to help you with your rehabilitation. Do you remember me?"

With a great effort to form his halting words, Zicheng said, "Face is familiar, I think you are friend, but I'm confused. Please tell me what happened to me. I need someone to explain. I feel a suture line on my head, so I think I have had brain surgery. I want to stand up." When Lishan rang the call button, the nurse appeared with a urinal. Zicheng shook his head. "Not in bed. Help me stand."

The two women helped him stand by the side of the bed. With the nurse holding the urinal, he relieved himself. They helped him back into bed.

Still having trouble speaking his words, he stammered, "Tell me now. What happened to me?"

"You had an operation to put your brain into a different body," Lishan answered. "You lost most of your old body in a car wreck."

"But where? Am I in China?"

"Your accident happened in Tibet, but you were brought to Chengdu, here in China. The surgery there saved your life but left you crippled. You elected to come here to Harbin, where Dr. Wong has perfected brain transplants," she explained.

"I'm a doctor, and I've never heard of brain transplants. Don't be ridiculous."

"It's a new procedure, and you're one of the first."

With a face reflecting anger, he replied, "I'm having trouble believing that. Let me think about it. Shortly after, his dinner tray arrived. "No," he said, shaking his head and closing his eyes.

"Zicheng, wake up. You have to eat," Lishan said sharply. He did not react. "Roger, wake up!" she said, emphasizing his American name. He responded with a start and a stare.

"I'm sorry," he mumbled, "Who am I?"

"You must remember; you are Wu Zicheng."

"I am Roger Scully."

"Forget Roger. We will not use that name again. Roger is dead."

She picked up the plastic tray from the bedside table. "Now, you're going to face the dinner challenge," she said. "Tonight, we will use a spoon and save the chopsticks for another day. First, try some juice." She steadied his cup and steered a straw to his mouth.

He sucked a mouthful of the amber liquid, then another. It looked like apple juice, but something was wrong. "No taste, no taste," as he frowned at the clear plastic spoon beside the white bowl.

"Try the porridge. You need the nourishment."

He waved his hands slowly over the bowl and spoon. Lishan, sensing his confusion, leaned forward and placed the spoon in his right hand. With a puzzled look, he changed it to his left hand.

"Zicheng, why are you changing hands?"

"Because I'm left-handed."

After a long pause, he plunged the utensil into the porridge and tried to guide it into his mouth. His hand trembled as he maneuvered the spoon. His first attempt hit his chin; his second attempt hit his cheek near his mouth. Food spattered his pillow.

Lishan kept an impassive face as she watched the struggle. The third try succeeded in hitting his open mouth but went too far in, and he gagged before he withdrew it enough to close his lips, clear the spoon, and swallow.

"Well done, Zicheng. Now try another spoonful." This time, he scooped the food, guided it to his mouth, and managed to eat it without a problem. A few swallows later, he paused.

"No taste."

"This food doesn't have much taste on its own. Next time they might put some meat on it."

With Lishan's assistance, he managed to eat almost half his dinner. It seemed strange to chew without flavor, although he could distinguish texture. As he struggled with the meal, he wondered about what was happening. He found the tasteless food depressing. *Am I here to die?* The familiar hospital surroundings reassured him, but it was not a hospital he knew. *Who are all these people?* The plastic spoon weighed like lead. Exhausted by the effort, he fell asleep without finishing the meal.

***

The next day, Roger smiled weakly when Lishan arrived, grinning with her ponytail swinging.

"Good morning, Zicheng. How are you today?"

"Not Zicheng. I am Roger. Are you going to tell me more about what happened to me?"

"As much as I know. Do you have any memory of why you had your operation?"

"None at all."

"You might find it hard to believe, but you had your brain transplanted into a different body."

"You told me that, but I find it ridiculous! I can't believe it."

"You'll understand when you have more recovery. But why don't we get you out of bed? The doctors want you to walk."

"Help me to the bathroom. Then I need to know more about this." His words were coming more easily now.

Lishan used the call button to bring the nurse. "It's not very far, and we'll help," she said. Lishan and the nurse helped Zicheng out of bed and supported him. He swayed from side to side until the nurse tightened her grip on his arm. *I have to move my feet. How do I do that?* After a pause, he slid his left foot forward a few inches. *Oh, I need to lift my feet.* Raising his right foot a few inches, he gingerly placed it six inches in front. He smiled at his accomplishment as he repeated the exercise for the ten-foot walk into his bathroom. By the time he reached the doorway, his gait was near-normal, albeit slow.

He glanced, then stared at the bathroom mirror. "What? Who is that?" he screamed. "What's going on?" Words came from the mouth of a bearded dark-haired man. He grimaced. "Agghhh. I am not that man. Is this a terrible trick?" Panic overwhelmed him; he grabbed the sides of the sink to steady himself as his body shook with a combination of fear and weakness. He wanted to call it another hallucination, like the frequently flashing lights.

"Calm down. Have your pee, and then I'll explain everything," said Lishan, with a tight grip on his arm. When he finished, they guided him back into bed, his face distorted with concern after another glance at the mirror where the vision of the bearded brown-eyed man destroyed his theory of having had a hallucination. He scowled at the two women.

He strained his weak voice, attempting to shout, "Who is that man in the mirror?"

"This will be a long story, but I'll try to fill you in on all the things you don't remember." Lishan spoke slowly but in a firm voice. "You were in a bad car accident in Tibet, and they airlifted you to the hospital in Chengdu. You had a severe crush injury, which forced the doctors there to perform a hemicorporectomy."

"A WHAT? I've never heard that term."

"It's a real term. About twenty-five of these procedures are in the medical literature." As she brought out her phone, she continued. "Here's your picture after the surgery in Chengdu. Dr. Wen and his team did it because your lower body was a pulpy mess. They had to remove your pelvis and hips." She displayed the picture.

His eyes opened wide at the sight of a naked and pale egg-shaped lower torso, with two lines of staples arcing up from the base to under his ribs at the sides. With a look of astonishment, he said, "Oh, my God! That was me? No legs? No balls and no dick? And that person has a colostomy. I don't have a colostomy!"

"You must try to remember, Zicheng."

"Roger," he said.

"No, not anymore. You have a new body now. New face, new body, new name. You are a new person."

"I don't understand you."

"You had many discussions with the Chengdu doctors about your future. You could not accept that you would always be in a wheelchair." With a proud smile, she continued, "Speaking of wheelchairs, let me show you a video of you before you came to Harbin."

She adjusted her phone for him to watch the screen. Through a blur, he saw a large, three-wheeled contraption lift his legless torso out of bed in a sling, then deposit the shortened body into a tub attached to the frame.

His face lit up as he recognized the blond man. "That's me, Roger Scully. I'm controlling that thing!" he said as the person pressed buttons and maneuvered the apparatus forward and backward, then in circles. He watched the device lift him out of the chair and place him back in bed. "Can I see that video again?"

Lishan replayed the video as he stared wide-eyed.

"Yes, that's the apparatus I designed to get you out of bed and mobile. It's not an ordinary wheelchair. See how your head is at eye level. I designed it for you. We called it the chariot because you sort of stood up in it."

"And you built it?"

"I designed it, and two technicians put it together. They had trouble taking orders from me, but I knew what I was doing."

"I have trouble believing that all that happened to me. That chariot thing worked?"

"Yes, it did. You were excited to get around the hospital, but within a few days, you pointed out it wouldn't get you out of a nursing home, let alone let you practice medicine. You were so depressed that you asked Dr. Wen in Chengdu to help you die."

"So, how'd I get here?"

"Dr. Wen told you that Dr. Wong, here in Harbin, had successfully transplanted a human brain. You came to Harbin to have your brain placed into a more functional body. And that's what has happened." Lishan waved her hand toward his toes. "You now have a different body but the same brain as before."

"I've never heard of such a procedure. You're making this up."

"You're the first person in the world to be alive after this transplant," she said, pointing to him.

"Where did they find a donor?"

"A prisoner condemned to die donated his body. You might find it confusing that your new body is not Caucasian, but there was no alternative donor. Before the surgery, the team here did many measurements and CT scans to help a physical anthropologist select a similar body-type donor. They then obliterated the donor's marrow with drugs and radiation. You donated your marrow to replace his."

"Wait a minute. I have my original marrow and not that of the donor?"

"Correct. The marrow swap was to lessen the likelihood of a rejection reaction against your brain. The surgery was successful." She laid her hand on his shoulder.

"So the new body explains my brown eyes instead of blue and my black hair instead of blond."

"Right, the doctors placed you in a cold coma for a few weeks to manage your post-operative care. Because they kept you cooled to protect your brain function, Dr. Wong calls it hypothermic hibernation. And now you're awake."

"But, I'm not Roger any more?"

"When you came here for the transplant program, they gave you the name Wu Zicheng to protect your confidentiality. When you lived in the hospital cottage getting ready for the surgery, we called you Zicheng. Only a few doctors know you were Roger Scully. You'll get used to being called Zicheng. Roger no longer exists."

Roger no longer existed. A revolting thought. He still felt like himself, and he was Roger. Wasn't he? "I'm going to be sick," he said as he turned on his side to vomit into the waiting basin.

The nurse stepped forward to wipe his face and mouth with a towel. He sat straighter in his bed and shook off the assistance.

"I'm sorry," Roger said, "I don't know what brought that on."

"Don't apologize. This experience must be an enormous shock."

"But tell me again, where did they get me a new body?"

"A prisoner condemned to death for crimes against the state donated his body. His family agreed to it as well. In China, that is quite common. The donor lives several months longer; he dies under an anesthetic instead of being shot."

"And where is my old body?"

"You donated your organs at the time of your surgery. You changed or saved the lives of seven other people when you donated your organs."

"So parts of Roger walk around in seven other people, and I am here as Zicheng. Is that correct?"

"You seem to understand that perfectly."

"And what is Zicheng supposed to do with his new body?"

"That is up to you. I'm only a medical student."

They were interrupted by a thin man, about age sixty, in orange scrubs and a white jacket. "Ni hao, Zicheng." The intruder whipped back the sheet from Zicheng's legs.

Lishan said, "This is your therapist to keep your skin and joints in condition." The man started massaging Zicheng's calves and then thighs. Zicheng recognized the kneading, rolling, and punching motions from his days in darkness. A few minutes later, Zicheng was face down on the bed, the therapist examining his buttocks for pressure sores. Lishan and the therapist exchanged a few words before the man's departure.

"He's a traditional therapist," Lishan explained. "He made sure you didn't get stiff joints or bed sores from your time in a coma. He will not be back; conventional physiotherapy will take over."

"But where do you come into my story? Your face and voice are familiar, but I don't know you."

"I'm your close friend, Zhou Lishan, and have been tending to you for months, both in Chengdu and here in Harbin. I'm a senior medical student, and I designed your chariot as my senior elective project. My undergraduate degree was in Mechanical Engineering. So, working with you, I got to know you. We fell in love and lived together for three months while they prepared you for your transplant."

He pointed to the plastic pitcher. "I need some water to keep talking. I'm not questioning your truthfulness, but where did this happen?"

She poured and handed him the water. "We lived in a cottage here on the hospital grounds with two other patients, Ke and Sung. We had a cook called Fong."

"My memory is like a jigsaw puzzle, and you just handed me a new piece." He could now picture their bedroom, its metal-framed hospital bed. Lishan had painted floral ivy on the posts, and he now remembered waking up one morning with the still-damp paint smeared on the back of his hand. How could he remember this now, when minutes ago, he would have sworn that no such thing had ever occurred?

He recalled Lishan's warmth next to him. He tingled with a feeling of love, remembered.

"Before the operation, you wrote an email to your parents about the planned surgery, and I promised to send it to them if the operation was successful. I did that yesterday. You should read the letter you sent them." She handed him a printout.

"It's too blurry. I can't read it."

She removed her large glasses and handed them to him. "Try these, and see if they help."

"I don't wear glasses."

"Maybe you do now. We'll get that checked." He waved off the glasses, and she replaced them on her nose. "I'll read it to you until we get your vision sorted out."

January 5

Dear Mom and Dad,

Happy New Year. I apologize for not telling you what is happening. I am not here in Harbin for prostheses to replace my missing legs. I am here to get a new body.

Yes, a new body. Tomorrow I will have my brain placed into another body. I have asked Lishan to send you this letter when I wake from my coma after the successful transplant. The post-op coma lasts for about two weeks, which explains why you have not heard from me. This letter confirms I am now awake and recovering from the surgery.

My surgeon, Dr. Wong, had done this procedure twice before, with success. I am planning to be his third medical triumph. I suggest you come and visit me here in Harbin. Understand that I will not look like the old Roger. Only the brain is the same. The face and body are new.

For many reasons, please keep my surgery secret. I still have to plan how to reintroduce Roger Scully to the world.

I could not have gone through the surgery without feeling confident of your love and support, which I still need. I hope you will be able to visit me soon in Harbin.

With much love,

Your son, Roger

Lishan smiled wanly back at Roger. "A few minutes after I sent the email, your parents called me. Of course, they were in a state of shock. I calmed them down when I told you you had survived the surgery well and were recovering. They've called me almost every six or eight hours since to confirm you are okay."

"So my parents know all about this?"

"They visited you in Chengdu. You told them you were coming to Harbin for a new kind of prosthesis. And they'll be coming here. We'll call them before they leave for the plane. They'll feel better when they know you're alive and talking."

Zicheng sat speechless for what seemed like minutes, with a dry mouth and open lips. Finally, he said, with effort, "That explains some things. My memory is slowly coming back. I know I was a doctor in Denver and going on a trip somewhere. I keep trying to place you. My brain seems scrambled."

"In Chengdu, you couldn't remember the accident or Tibet. The doctors explained that it was retrograde amnesia from a concussion. Quite common. Nobody could predict what your memory would be like after the transplant because you're the first survivor of this procedure. You—"

Roger interrupted in a loud voice, "What do you mean I'm the first survivor? Were they experimenting on me?"

She nodded. "I guess you can consider the transplant as an experiment, but it worked.

You don't seem to remember Chengdu. Do you recall anything about your months here in Harbin before this surgery?"

"Almost nothing, but you're helping me with that. I remember you next to me in bed." He wondered why he felt such an attraction to this student. What was the past?

"We had some good times together in those months. I have good memories, and you seem like the same man I fell in love with. Maybe your memories will return. That would be nice."

He gasped. "I need to lie down. The flashes and the hiss have started up again." As he laid back, he covered his eyes with his hands. She adjusted his pillows, cranked down the bed, and kissed the back of his hands as he lay sobbing.

17

She kissed his forehead. "Try to sleep, Zicheng. I have to be at my clinic for appointments. I'll be back soon."

Lishan returned just after his tasteless dinner. He noticed she was attractive, about the right weight for her five-foot-five body. The sweater under her student jacket covered small but pert breasts. A straight black skirt and white sneakers completed the outfit.

"We should call your parents now. It'll be early morning in Boston, but they should still be at home." He hesitated, knowing it would be a difficult conversation, but Lishan handed him his phone after she entered the Boston number.

Before he knew what was happening, his mother's voice was on the other end.

"Mom," he said. "It's Roger."

She gasped, "Roger?" and he realized she did not recognize his voice. Of course, she didn't. "Are you really Roger, or is this some terrible joke?"

"It's me, Mom. The operation changed my voice."

"If you're Roger, then you know our cat's name."

"Pharaoh." He envisioned the large calico cat on its usual perch on the kitchen counter.

"Oh my God, Roger. I'm so glad to hear from you. I've been worried sick."

"I'm sorry, Mom. It's my first chance to call you since just before my surgery. He spoke briefly to both his mother and father, trying to summarize what he had undergone. He stumbled with many words and had to repeat sentences. The anxiety in their voices told him they couldn't quite comprehend the situation.

"Mom, I'll have Lishan send you a picture right away. Just don't get upset when I look so different. I'm still the same Roger, and remember how horrible I must have looked in Chengdu." Roger

18

recalled Lishan's Chengdu photograph. His new appearance was an improved body, but how would his parents accept a son with no resemblance to his former self?

"But how are you feeling? Do you have pain? Are you out of bed?"

"I'm doing well, with no real pain. I'm starting to walk around and getting physiotherapy. I'm a different person than when you saw me in Chengdu. Don't worry. I'm making a good recovery."

"We have a flight today, but it takes two days to get to Harbin. We've been so worried about you, and we couldn't seem to contact you. Oh, God. We're so relieved. We'll see you in a few days. Is there anything we can bring?"

"Yeah, bring me a Red Sox cap, Mom. I love you."

He wondered if the conversation had been as trying for them as it had been for him. That night, as usual, Zicheng had dreams so real that he felt he was still in them when he awoke. He was doing his residency; he was working in Denver. In his most vivid experience, he was hiking with Joanne on a bright winter day. When they arrived at the frozen pond, they sat on a log to put on their skates. He awoke still smelling the fresh mountain air and hearing Joanne's laugh as they skated. His dreams were filling in more of his jigsaw memory.

"Good morning, Zicheng. Do you remember me?" asked the tall doctor striding into the sunlit room.

"You seem familiar, but my memory's not too good at the moment." Zicheng's words were slow as he worked to enunciate his thoughts.

"I'm Peter Bin, your psychiatrist. We talked a lot before your surgery. I've been trying to help you wake up and recover from the coma. Do you know where you are?"

"Someone told me, Harbin, in China."

"Do you know the date?"

"I haven't a clue. Because I see snow outside, I assume it's winter."

"Let's talk about your memory. Tell me your life history."

"I've been trying to remember my life, but everything is patchy. I grew up in Boston. I played hockey in high school at Boston Latin. I'm having trouble remembering college and medical school, except for the first day in med school. We paraded into the anatomy lab, where I met my cadaver on the dissecting table. The four of us were all nervous when we opened the metal cover of the table. We pulled back a damp cloth to see this skinny old dead person with yellowish skin. I even remember the smell of embalming fluid in a reservoir at the foot of the table. Two fabric wicks ran alongside the body from the reservoir to preserve the body for the months of dissection. I don't know why I can remember that so clearly."

"That's a moment every doctor remembers. A major event is more likely to reappear in your memory early."

"I keep remembering Joanne, my wife. I remember her illness, the months of treatment, and her death and burial. It's the most upsetting of my dreams and recollections. And then things kind of go blank."

"You're doing remarkably well. With amnesia like this, most of the blanks will fill in with time. You were taking Mandarin lessons before your surgery. Can you remember any of it?"

"That's funny. I understand some of the words I hear and wonder why. I'm sure I never learned Mandarin in Boston."

"I'm delighted with your recovery; I'll visit every few days. The other doctors will take care of any physical needs. We'll talk more another day. I see one of your therapists waiting."

The physiotherapist (PT) was first. Initially, she measured the angles of his limb movements, then estimated strength. With her hands near his shoulders, she had him stand with feet close together. He wobbled slightly.

"Now, close your eyes."

She grasped his shoulders when his sudden swaying started a fall. Zicheng had failed the balance test. Although the PT could not speak English, she was able to communicate with him through gestures. At the end of an hour of assessment, he wanted to get back to bed. However, the occupational therapist (OT) was already waiting.

The OT, also non-English speaking, had him do activities such as placing various pegs in holes, arranging playing cards in order, and picking items from a tray. He found all the tasks difficult, if not impossible. His heavily-calloused fingers flexed poorly to his command. He could understand her orders, but he lacked coordination. He also had trouble gripping the pegs of the puzzle; he could not judge size. The OT refused his request to help him back to bed.

Another attendant was waiting with a wheelchair.

"Now what?" Roger asked.

"Audiology," she said as she assisted him into the chair to push him to her laboratory.

Tired but resigned, Roger tolerated almost an hour of hearing clicks, whistles, and voices. Finally, as he was about to protest, the technician explained his results.

"If you look at the audiograms before and after your surgery, you see that your hearing has improved. When we tested you before, we found a pattern of noise-induced hearing loss. My notes say that you knew about it and blamed it on playing in a rock band."

Another piece of the jigsaw puzzle clicked into place. "Oh, yeah. Too many rim shots by the drummer. But why am I better?"

"You have new ears now."

"That's a hell of a way to improve my hearing. What about the hissing I always hear?"

"I think it's irritation of the nerve giving you tinnitus. It should go away with time."

His bed beckoned. He refused to eat dinner and slept through the rest of the afternoon and night. In his dreams, he was a Chinese man speaking Mandarin in Boston, with no one understanding his requests for assistance.

The following morning, Doctors Wong and Li were pleased to watch the end of the OT session. The older man, nodding approval, said, "I am Doctor Wong. Are you having any pain?"

"A bit of a headache, but it's getting better."

They examined his incision lines before Li began his neurologic assessment. "Rub your right heel on your left shin. Now the other foot. Close your eyes and touch your nose. Let's see you stand up." He helped Roger to his feet.

Knees shaking, Roger said, "I don't do this too well."

Li nodded approval. "You will get there soon. You're remarkable. The world will have trouble believing this."

When they left, Roger thought about his medical team. They seemed very serious but lacking in any apparent warmth or concern. He laid back and fell asleep.

"Ni hao ma, Zicheng!" Lishan woke him up with her greeting.

"Tired, very tired," he said, with some difficulty forming the words.

"Major surgery always leaves you tired. You're learning to use your body all over again. I met with both the PT and OT just before I came here. They're optimistic; all your muscles are working and well-controlled. Remember, your body donor was in excellent physical shape, so that is to your benefit. Strength and coordination will come with therapy. Both therapists will be back every day. And I'm here to work with you, too," Lishan said. "I have a favorite expression: The last leg of a journey just marks the halfway point."

"Were you reading *Love Story* to me when I was out cold?"

"Yes, that was me."

"Why were you doing that?"

"Dr. Bin, the psychiatrist, told us that so-called unconscious people often report hearing things while they are in a coma. Before your surgery, I asked you what I should read to you during the coma, and you suggested *Love Story* as a book you could relate to because of losing your wife."

"My wife, Joanne." He saw an ice rink and their breath in the cold air. Joanne was laughing. Or crying? He tried to shake off this piece of the jigsaw.

"I don't think I can walk to the john alone. Can you get help?"

Lishan called a nurse. They got him to the bathroom, and he had another look at a man called Zicheng. He gazed in the mirror for several minutes. He had to get used to a different face and hair that was a black, straight two-week stubble instead of blond and curly locks. His thick dark eyebrows were a distinct change from his previous almost-white ones. He scowled at the full beard and decided that it would have to go. He noticed he was now a circumcised man, a change from before. *Must have been a Muslim donor.* From somewhere, he remembered that the Chinese did not circumcise most male infants. He looked at his now prominent Adam's apple; the larger size might explain the deep baritone voice that had replaced his previous reedy tenor. His change in eye color did not bother him.

"Lishan, I need to shave off this beard, but I'll need help."

"You're not strong enough to stand at the sink. I'll get one of the hospital people to shave you in bed." Lishan and the nurse helped him back to the bed. A few minutes later, the nurse returned with a male attendant for whom Lishan translated Roger's wish to have no beard or mustache.

After, when Lishan held up a mirror, Roger said, "I see a slight improvement. I guess I have to learn to live with my new face." He continued to examine his appearance, looking in vain for Roger's features, except for eyes, which were similar in shape but brown rather than blue.

That afternoon, Lishan announced, "Okay, time for you to get dressed."

"What? Why?"

"You're not going to live in a hospital gown for the rest of your life. You should be in clothes when your parents arrive tomorrow afternoon."

"I have no clothes."

"Oh, yes, you do. While you were waking up, I went shopping. You now have underwear, jeans, a shirt, shoes, and socks." She fetched an armful of clothes from his closet.

"How did you know the size?"

"Dr. Li gave me a list of sizes from the donor."

"How am I going to pay you for this?"

"In Chengdu, when I met your parents, your father gave me $300 to use for any of your incidental expenses."

Her repeated references to Chengdu were filling in some of the missing puzzle pieces. He recalled his parents visiting at his bedside, a flash of his mother in tears. He recalled the desolation of being without a complete body. It was like losing himself, like losing Joanne. He remembered.

He left his thoughts of Joanne to return his attention to Lishan and the clothing. Zicheng was relieved that he would not be wearing a dead man's clothes.

"Brand new," said Lishan.

He stared at the assortment of clothing. *I should know how to put these on.* He picked up the buttoned and folded shirt. His fingers failed to free any buttons from the holes. Lishan stepped up and undid all the buttons. His attempt at dressing was awkward. He leaned against the bed and tried to pull on his jockey shorts under his hospital gown. When he almost fell over, Lishan giggled and lifted each foot into the shorts before she pulled them up.

"Well, I guess I have no secrets from you."

"Nothing I haven't seen before."

Arms and legs refused to cooperate. Lishan watched the struggle after he waved her away and finally got into his shirt and jeans. He made only one attempt at the shirt buttons and jeans zipper before motioning her closer.

"This is embarrassing. I'm like a little boy that needs his mother to dress him."

"Don't worry about it. You have to relearn all the things you take for granted. I love helping you."

The next test was his attempt to tie his sneaker laces. After repeated fumbling failures, Lishan leaned forward to assist.

"No, I have to do it myself, and I will," Zicheng insisted. Seated, he succeeded on his next attempt.

"There you go." Then in a sing-song voice like a childhood nursery rhyme, she sang, "Try and fail; try and fail, then try and tie." They laughed together.

Lishan left for one of her clinical assignments. From standing alone, Zicheng shuffled carefully to the bathroom. Gazing at his reflection in the mirror, he decided he looked better shaved and dressed. However, he still felt as though he was watching a stranger. His brain spun slowly. *Is that Roger Scully?*

CHAPTER 3

Mildred and Walter Scully entered the room timidly, Walter first putting his head through the doorway.

"Come in, Dad. I won't bite."

With startled faces, they entered to stare at the man sitting in the armchair, dressed in jeans and a flannel shirt. "Yes, it's me," he said.

Mildred walked toward him with tentative steps. "Roger, really?"

"I look and sound different, but isn't it a big improvement since you last saw me? I'm still me, Mom. Remember the kid who got hot chocolate after hockey practice."

She rushed toward him, hugged him, and kissed him. "Oh my God, Roger. I worried I would never see you alive again. Let me get used to you. I'm glad you got rid of that beard you had in the picture." She stood back and stared as tears trickled down her cheeks.

Roger quivered slightly at the familiar scent of his mother's lilac perfume. He struggled to his feet, needing to feel his mother's embrace. At age thirty-nine, he still wanted his mother's love. His knees were going to rubber; he quickly sat back in the chair. She opened her purse and handed him the Red Sox cap.

With a grin, Roger put on the cap. It covered many of the suture lines visible through the stubble on his scalp. "Perfect fit."

Walter stepped forward and shook his son's hand. "You're a miracle. This is a happy day. We came here as soon as we could. We just dropped our bags at the hotel and kept the same taxi."

"I'm glad you're here. Now I feel more like myself. How are the Bruins doing?"

"Leading the conference at the moment," his father said.

Feeling sudden fatigue, Roger suggested, "You can't believe how tired I get. I need to sleep a bit. You should go back to your hotel and get some rest. You're on a twelve-hour time change. We'll have lots of time to talk tomorrow. They don't enforce any visiting hours here."

"You're not going to get rid of us that quick. I'm going to just sit here and look at you for a while," Mildred said.

"I agree with your mom. When we left you in Chengdu, I thought we would never see you alive again. We flew out of Boston as soon as we heard about the Tibet accident. We had never even heard of Chengdu.

"We got there just before you had that awful surgery. Dr. Wen shocked us when he told us what they had done. Mom fainted in the waiting room; I wasn't much better. I was angry that they had not warned us. I shouted at the surgeon, which was wrong. After the operation, you looked like shit, to put it mildly.

"We stayed until you were moved from the ICU into a regular hospital ward, with those three other patients. That's where we met Lishan. You're lucky she's been looking out for you ever since the surgery. We appreciate her efforts, and the chariot was an inspired invention."

"It got me out of bed and mobile, but it wasn't a long-term solution. At least for me."

His parents' discussion fit into Lishan's account of Chengdu. He recalled them standing at his bedside after the hemicorporectomy.

"I feel like a newborn who has to become an adult in a few weeks."

"Until we heard about this transplant, I worried that you'd kill yourself instead of coming home." As Walter Scully spoke, he gestured hopelessness as his eyes filled with tears. Pulling himself erect, he said, "We have to get you out of this place as soon as we can."

After twenty minutes of discussion about his strength, voice, therapy, and memory, Roger was fading. With weak smiles and after several hugs, the Scullys departed. Roger slipped out of his clothes, got into his bed, and drifted into a strange sleep. He dreamed of his childhood dog and playing hockey, eating with Joanne. He woke in the night and lay alone in the dark, missing those things. His planned life had disappeared with his old body. Beloved, but gone. He could never go home; it would never be the same.

When the Scullys arrived the next morning, Lishan was visiting. Mildred remembered her from Chengdu and hugged her tightly. "You've been so good to Roger. Thank you for all you have done."

"It's been my pleasure. I'll let you visit. I have to be going to my clinical duties, and I can see you later." She patted Roger on the arm and left quickly.

"I'm sorry I keep staring, but it's just too hard to believe. Tell us more about the surgery and what they did," said Mildred.

Zicheng talked about his satisfaction with the surgery and his progress with the PT and OT. "I'm working hard to get my strength back. I've started walking in the hall, and I intend to go further each day. Dad, if you don't mind me taking your arm, let's do that walk now," he said as he stood up with shaky knees.

His father grabbed his son's arm, looking frightened at the responsibility. After a pause, the pair shuffled to the door, turned, and disappeared down the corridor. Mildred followed close behind with a look of concern.

"We'll go to the first door, Dad. Tomorrow will be the second door."

When they returned, Roger headed for the bed, not the chair. His father helped him onto the bed and removed his sneakers.

"Thanks, Dad. I'm not quite as strong as I thought."

"You'll do well. I know your determination and spirit. Can I help you take off your clothes?"

"No thanks, just let me nap, and someone will help me later. You should go now."

Roger slept until a nurse awakened him for his late afternoon pill. Although he struggled, he undressed without assistance. He appreciated the new pajamas that had come with his other clothes. Lishan reappeared, as usual, at dinner time.

"Well, how did the visit go today?"

"They're beginning to accept their newborn son. Dad helped me walk in the hallway. Mom mostly stared at me with the strangest smile that never left her face. They'll be back tomorrow. I'm still tired from their visit. How was your day?"

"Busy as usual. A lot of this clinical clerkship is cheap, forced labor. You know, preadmission histories, drawing blood, and all the usual shit. Tonight, they expect me to volunteer in the ER, where they're always understaffed. If I'm lucky, they'll let me suture up a few drunks."

"Been there, done that. You bring back my memories of med school and internship. I remember my first time drawing blood, the first time I sutured a live person." More pieces in the jigsaw puzzle.

When his dinner tray arrived, Lishan watched him manipulate his utensils.

"Hey, you're getting along fast in feeding yourself."

"But chicken feet in porridge is not appealing. I never liked porridge, and I find chicken feet revolting."

"You said the same thing when we lived in the cottage. You finally persuaded Fong, the cook, to prepare more Western food. You enjoyed some of the Szechuan dishes in Chengdu, didn't you?"

He suddenly remembered the spicy and hot noodles he had enjoyed in a room with three other patients. They had taught him the challenging game of Go.

"Yes, I remember. And you and I played Go some evenings. I even beat you once."

"You're just making that up," she teased with a smile. "Would you like me to bring over the game from the cottage?"

"It would be a good form of OT if I can pick up and place the tiles with my clumsy fingers."

"I'll have it for tomorrow night. I'll be off-call then. But I better go and get my supper before I have to be in the ER."

She leaned over the bed, attempting to kiss his cheek. He caught her head, turned it, and kissed her lips. She repeated the kiss and left with a broad smile. After dinner, Zicheng fell asleep thinking of Lishan and recalling his love for her before the surgery.

When his parents returned the next morning, they watched Roger work with the PT. They commented to each other about their son's energy and determination in performing the various routines. After the PT, the OT appeared immediately. Mildred watched him place pegs in holes and shouted, "Way to go, Rog," when he succeeded. She then covered her mouth with a look of embarrassment. Roger grinned at her encouragement.

As the OT departed, Roger turned to his parents. "Look, I always need a nap after all this. Why don't you find lunch and then come back? I'd like Dad to help me again with my walking."

After she kissed her son once again, Mildred and Walter waved goodbye and strolled out the door, hand in hand. When they returned an hour later, Roger was finishing his lunch in his chair.

"Perfect timing, Dad. I slept about twenty minutes. I want to try the walk again. Today we'll go to the second door. Watch me get out of the chair." With that, he rolled forward slightly and sprang to his feet without using his arms. Once erect, he staggered somewhat but waved off his father's arm and stabilized his stance. "The PT taught me that the first day, and I've been practicing it every chance I get. This was the first time I did it without using any arms at all. Even if I get tired, I'm glad to be out of bed. I never understood that bed rest is worse than living in a cage. And now I'm free!"

"I remember teaching you to skate on the backyard rink I made. You insisted on getting up early to practice almost every day. I've always been proud of your determination. Now let's try the walk."

Today's walk, again observed by Mildred, was twice the length of the previous days.

After a short chat about the Bruin's chances for the Stanley Cup, Roger was ready to explain his name change. "If you noticed the name on my chart or my wrist band, it says Wu Zicheng. No mention of Roger Scully. When I arrived here, they gave me this Chinese name to protect my confidentiality. Now they insist on calling me Zicheng, and if you ask any questions about me, you might need to use that name instead of Roger Scully."

Both parents frowned. Walter spoke up. "I don't like that at all. Those Chinese foreigners can't take away your name. I'm going to protest."

"Easy, dad. Don't sound like a racist Boston Southie. The name's only a temporary thing while I'm in the hospital. I found it hard at first, but now I'm used to being called Zicheng. I like it when you call me Roger, so don't change that."

"When you explain it that way, my Irish temper tends to go down, but there's nothing wrong with being a Southie. To us, you will always be Roger Scully."

"Don't sweat the name. Realize how far I've come. I had no chance for a successful or independent life when you saw me in Chengdu." His parents quickly glanced at each other, recalling how the sight of his truncated body had devastated them when they visited China. "Be happy for me. Appreciate that the doctors here have given me a second life, one where I will be independent. I might even get back to being a doctor again."

"Oh my God, that would be wonderful. We're so grateful for your surgery," his mother said. "It's just that we were so confused and anxious about what was happening to you, and when we didn't hear anything for over two weeks, that made it worse."

"Yes, I know, and I'm sorry about that. One thing you probably didn't notice—my transplant was on what would have been Joanne's birthday. I'll always remember January sixth as the day of her birth and the day of my re-birth, as it were. A few days ago, I didn't remember her death, but my memory is filling in fast."

"Oh, my, we never thought of the date," his mom sighed. "So, what happens next? When can you come home?"

"I've got several months of treatment before I'm ready to travel. You can see I'm doing well, but I'm still pretty weak, and I still need a lot of physio and OT. I'm also on a drug that's only available here. Don't worry. You'll see me soon enough. I'm hoping that soon I'll move back to the cottage where I lived, waiting for the surgery. But for now, I think it's time for you to go home."

"My goodness, we've just arrived, and you want to get rid of us."

"Well, I don't think there's anything to interest you in Harbin. You can see I'm doing fine, so you can get back to running the restaurant. I'll come home as soon as I can. In the meantime, promise me you won't tell anyone about my surgery and transplant. Let's keep most of this secret for now. Just tell people I'm getting a new kind of prosthesis for my missing legs."

His father replied, "Whatever you say, this one's your call. We love you, no matter what you look like. We just need a little time to get used to having a son who looks Chinese. It's difficult to absorb the reality of all these amazing things that have happened to you. I'll feel better when you're back in Natick, where you belong."

His mother finally smiled, "It's going to be wonderful, getting your health back."

Walter had been working his phone and soon announced, "We can book a flight for Monday morning to Hong Kong and then on to Boston. I think we should take it because the next available reservation would be a week later."

Mildred frowned while Roger spoke up, "Take it, Dad. You don't want to sit around here for weeks." They continued to watch his PT and OT treatment for the next few days. Walks lengthened, smiles abounded. On Monday, after an early morning visit, the parents left Harbin. Although they promised not to share the images, they had loaded their phones with pictures of them with their new son.

CHAPTER 4

At 2 a.m., his teeth chattered while uncontrollable shivering and a violent headache broke his sleep. Sweat poured from his forehead and face. *Am I dying?* Then he recognized a rigor. He struggled to reach the call button and finally summoned the nurse. Twenty minutes later, Dr. Li appeared. He heard the nurse say, "When I came in, I thought the bed would walk across the room. His temp was 39 Celsius. Pulse 140 and blood pressure 120 over 80. That's why I called to get you out of bed. I started the IV without an order."

"Good work. Crank up his IV to full and get 200 mg Solumedrol for a stat dose. And get a blood sample to the lab for culture, white count, and diff. Zicheng, do you hurt anywhere?"

"Just my head."

Li put his hand under Zicheng's head and flexed it forward. "Did that make it worse?"

"No."

"No sign of meningeal irritation, then." He continued to examine Zicheng, paying close attention to heart and lungs. "I already put in a call for Amy Chu. Some aspirin will take your temp down until the steroids start to work."

When immunologist Dr. Amy Chu arrived, still in her fur coat, Li summarized the history and findings, then said, "I'm concerned that he might have meningitis, which could be bacterial or, and we hope not, fungal. I'd feel better if we did a spinal tap to rule out meningitis."

Zicheng was listening intently to their discussion of his problem. His body ached from the strenuous shaking a few hours earlier. He would never forget the end-of-the-world feeling. A nurse had called Lishan at the cottage. She now stood by his bed, holding his hand, her lips pursed as she concentrated on the conversation.

Doctor Chu spoke up, "I think we're dealing with a rejection problem. I agree with doing the spinal tap, but we'll continue treating the possible rejection. First, we will use steroids and then consider our next line of defense. Give him another 100 mg of Solumedrol IV stat. I'm going to the lab to look at the white cell morphology and get the hematology results. In the meantime, keep him cool and well hydrated until we have some answers." With that, she rushed out, her long coat billowing behind her long strides.

Li now approached Zicheng. "I think you heard us talking. Your temperature and rigors are almost certainly due to a rejection reaction, but I'll do a spinal tap to rule out meningitis. Do you understand?"

"Yeah. Remember, I'm still a doctor. Can this reaction kill me?"

"It's possible but unlikely." In the transplant business, we get used to rejection crises. You'll feel crappy for the rest of the day and may have another rigor or two before the steroids kick in, but you'll feel much better tomorrow.

A nurse entered, carrying a towel-covered tray. She helped Zicheng to lie on his side, spine near the edge of the bed. "Bring your knees up near your chest," she said.

Li swabbed the back and deftly inserted a needle attached to a three-way valve and vertical glass tube. "Record normal 200 mm pressure," he said to the nurse, then flipped the stopcock, filled the syringe from the vertical cylinder, and withdrew the needle. The nurse was ready with a bandage. He handed the fluid specimen to Lishan and said, "Run this to the lab for stat analysis and culture."

Lishan's hands shook as she took the test tube. She ran from the room without comment. Less than ten minutes later, she returned, her face composed into a stoical expression. Her arched eyebrows asked Li a question.

"Lishan, it's okay. We're dealing with a common complication. He's in no danger at the moment."

"I don't want to leave him. If I sleep on his couch tonight, will someone kick me out?"

"No, it's a good idea. We won't need to have a special nurse with him overnight."

Zicheng was relieved to lie back down. He closed his eyes and dozed. Within an hour, Dr. Chu reappeared. "Okay, Zicheng, the good news is that you don't have a meningeal infection. The other news is that you are experiencing a rejection phenomenon. We had hoped to prevent this, but we did not, so now we'll treat it. We're ahead of the Americans on this problem because we have a more aggressive and better-organized transplant program. You'll get IV medications for the next few days, but after that, you'll have a combination of daily pills and occasional needle sticks. You won't feel much better for the rest of today, but by tomorrow you should notice a big improvement."

Lishan had been watching and listening intently. When the doctors left, she pulled her chair to the bedside, took Zicheng's hand, and said, "That's great news about no meningitis. I don't know much about immune reactions. A professor discussed the topic in one of my medical school lectures, but I've no clinical experience in that area."

"Don't worry about that. You're not my doctor."

Throughout the day, Zicheng had several rigors, each one leaving him exhausted. The final one occurred about 5 p.m., and an hour later, he started to feel better—the steroids were working. With Lishan's assistance, he managed a large glass of apple juice and another glass of high-protein drink.

"My God, I tasted the apple juice for the first time. I never thought I would appreciate apple juice, the most hated drink in the hospital."

"Dear, you're getting better already. They tell me you'll start on a new special antirejection drug that should be here in the next hour. How do you feel?"

In a weary voice, Zicheng replied, "I feel like I've been through a food blender. I ache all over, but most of my headache's gone. If they let me alone, I think I'll fall asleep."

"I'll tell the nurses not to disturb you for a while." She kissed his cheek, and he fell asleep. Throughout the night, he was awakened every two hours by nurses checking his vital signs. The sight of Lishan asleep on his couch produced a feeling of warm confidence.

In the morning, Zicheng felt much better. He was glad to see his breakfast, especially the orange juice he was beginning to taste. Lishan watched while Dr. Chu and Dr. Li read his chart. "You're a better man today than yesterday," Li concluded. "The combination of drugs is working. If all goes well today, we'll transfer you back to your cottage tomorrow. How does that sound?"

"I'd like that. Is there any way we can stop having my vitals taken every few hours?"

"We can take care of that," Li replied.

"Are you sure I am having a rejection problem?"

Chu responded, "We're pretty sure of that. We're using steroids, cyclosporine, and a new antirejection drug that I developed. It's doing very well in its clinical trials, and I think it'll be good for you. You responded very quickly to our treatment, but we'll keep a careful eye on you." The two doctors departed, leaving him alone with Lishan.

"Thank you for spending the night here with me. Very sweet, and I think I'm falling in love with you again," Zicheng said.

A wide smile and fully-opened eyes covered most of Lishan's face as she approached him. "I'm glad to hear that. I was worried that you had forgotten me. Right now, I have to attend rounds, but I'll be back soon. I love you, Roger." She squeezed his hand and started to leave.

He halted her exit with a firm voice. "Lishan, you have to be more careful. Remember, I am now Zicheng, and we are not to use the name Roger again." He laughed, "Don't I look like a Zicheng?" She smiled back, kissed him on the lips, and left with a wave. He rang for help to get out of bed, then, clutching the IV pole, shuffled to the bathroom. Exiting under the nurse's watchful eye, he walked the IV pole to the corridor and back. "I've got to get my strength back," he explained. "Spending weeks mostly in bed has made me a total wimp." He didn't like the word "wimp" and made an ugly face when he said it. His physical strength had always been a source of pride for him, and to now inhabit a somewhat flabby body with weak limbs made him irritable. After lunch, he took another short walk and then rested in the armchair. Lishan was surprised to see him sitting in his chair, fully dressed, eating dinner when she returned.

"Wow, you're getting better fast," she exclaimed. "What do the doctors say?"

"They plan on sending me back to the cottage tomorrow, so I guess I'll be off of the IV by then. They'll monitor me closely, but I should be independent. I want to get back in shape to start living that new life they promised. You're part of that life."

"That's nice to hear. Ke and Sung will be glad to see you. Do you remember them?"

"Ah, no. Remind me."

"They're two men who volunteered for the same surgery you had. You lived with them for three months and became good friends. They're like you. They see nothing to live for in their present condition, so they volunteered for the transplant program. When you see them, try to recognize them. Ke has a lot of burn scarring on his head and neck with a strange voice; Sung is in a wheelchair with spina bifida. I'm sure they'll understand that your memory is still coming back, but they'll be delighted at how well the operation worked. I hear that one of them will get his operation soon. Got to run now. I was lucky to get my clinical clerkship transferred here from Chengdu, but it's a lot of work." Lishan smiled and left to take care of other responsibilities.

Lishan's description of Ke and Sung flooded his brain with new memories. Ke's strange belched voice after a fire destroyed his larynx. Sung, all his life in a wheelchair, but a history of creating action programs for Visual Reality (VR). All three were victims of various tragedies with a unique solution that created strong bonds. Zicheng visualized the cottage interior, his bedroom, and Lishan next to him in bed. The jigsaw was filling in rapidly from its solid edges.

Soon after, Dr. Chu came in, looking serious. "Zicheng, we're going to change plans. Your afternoon bloodwork showed a drop in your hematocrit. I discussed it with our hematologist, and we suspect that hemolysis is destroying some of your red cells; this is a well-known problem in transplants, but we had hoped to avoid it with you.

"We'll add one more medication and watch your bloodwork. You have one asset that most transplant patients lack. We've an ample supply of blood we took from your previous body. That means we can transfuse you at any time with no danger. However, we need to monitor your kidney functions, so you're going to be here a few extra days. Do you understand?"

"Damn, that's a setback," Zicheng groaned. "I guess I just have to deal with it." He chastised himself for being so optimistic. As a doctor, he was well aware of the multiple complications that can occur after major surgery.

"We're going to measure your intake and output, Zicheng," Chu cautioned, "so make sure you do what the nurses tell you for the next few days. And don't worry, we're going to get you through this hiccup."

Shortly after Chu's departure, the rigors returned. Same shivering, sweating, and suffering as the first one. Zicheng lay tired, depressed, and soaking wet. And he had thought he was in the clear.

Lishan returned as they were changing his damp sheets. He shared the news about the latest rigor and the need to stay in the hospital for a few more days. Concern lined her face. "Oh, that's too bad. I'm sure you'll do well. I'll sleep here again tonight to keep an eye on you. Is there anything I can get you for the next few days?"

"Yeah, a fully recovered body. Got any spare ones around? Maybe I got a bad one on the first try."

"I don't find that funny, but I'm glad you're getting better. What can I get you?"

"If I have the laptop, I could continue working on the Chinese characters, but I might have trouble reading anything up close."

"I'll mention it to Doctor Li, and he'll arrange an ophthalmology consult. Your reading is important. Get back into bed and rest. The clean sheets will feel good."

"I'm exhausted. I'll brush my teeth and go to bed." He stood up to kiss and hug her briefly before she left. He was surprised to feel aroused as they touched. However, he was so tired that he was soon asleep.

On one of his routine morning visits, Dr. Li sat down and said, "I think we need to talk about your name. Lishan tells me you're not happy with Wu Zicheng."

"That's correct. I'm Roger Scully."

"When you transferred in here from Chengdu, we created a new name to ensure your confidentiality, in keeping with our policy for any new patients coming into the experimental surgery unit. In your stay here, including the time at the cottage, we have always referred to you as Zicheng.

Zicheng nodded his understanding.

Li continued, "When we did your transplant, a surgical team stripped your body of its other organs to use in other patients. Do you understand that?"

"I understand."

"The remaining corpse was sent to the morgue for cremation. That body carried the toe tag of Roger Scully."

Zicheng blanched at the image described. He felt his stomach drop before his muscles tightened. He nodded his understanding.

Li placed his right hand over Zicheng's. "Now you understand the situation. For us, Roger Scully is dead. Wu Zicheng is our patient. I suggest you accept your new identity and enjoy it."

"I see your point, but it'll take some getting used to."

Li stood up to leave and offered his hand to Zicheng. As they shook hands, he added, "This identity change is the most difficult part of your psychologic recovery. Good luck with it. If our team can help you in any way, don't hesitate to ask us."

"Thank you for your kind explanation. I'll do my best."

Notwithstanding Zicheng's occasional shaking and his additional medications, the occupational therapist still visited daily. She had him perform simple tasks concerned with touch and feel and finger dexterity; each day showed improvement. Visual disturbances lessened. When he had first awakened from his coma, flashing lights disturbed every image. The lights were fewer now, distorting his vision less. Li explained that in the donor's eyes, retinal rods relayed light signals as electrical impulses to the back of Zicheng's head, but his brain had to relearn the meaning of those impulses. Similarly, his hearing was improving as the waterfall noise diminished.

The following day after the usual routine of vital signs and blood draw, Zicheng was surprised to see the IV nurse carrying a plastic bag of blood. Without comment, she hooked up the blood to his IV, adjusted the flow, and left. Shortly after, Dr. Chu came in and explained to Zicheng, "We could probably get by without giving you blood, but your hematocrits down a bit, and we want to boost your strength to hasten your recovery. Any more rigors?"

"Not since last evening. I'm sleeping well, except for the damn nurses and the phlebotomist coming in at 5 a.m. My headache is gone, so I'm ready to go." He made a move as if getting out of bed.

"Not quite yet," Chu cautioned. "Your urinary output is good, and I'll have your renal function tests back in another hour or so. I won't keep you in this part of the hospital any longer than necessary. As you know, hospitals are not the safest of places, and you'll be better off living in your cottage."

"Thank you for your understanding. You're treating me very well here. I know you're not the person who can improve the food," he laughed.

Shortly after, Dr. Tsen, the ophthalmology resident, appeared. She introduced herself and started questions about his previous eye history. Lishan interrupted, "You don't understand. Zicheng is in another person's body. These are not his original eyes."

Tsen looked puzzled. Zicheng watched Lishan take ten minutes to brief her on the transplant story. Agog, Tsen responded. "Wow, never heard of anything like that. Well, let's help you out. Can you get to the eye exam room?"

Lishan spoke up. "He can walk a little, but let's use the wheelchair, and we'll follow you."

Twenty minutes of testing and examination in the ophthalmology department produced a lens prescription. Dr. Tsen explained, "They can fill this next door. It's a simple refractive error you were born with—oh, I guess I got mixed up, but you know what I mean. It was a pleasure to meet you. Good luck in your new life." She escorted them to the optician's office next door. Ten minutes later, they left with the promise that Zicheng's new glasses would arrive later that day. But Zicheng was still hearing the ophthalmologist's words, "Good luck in your new life." *Was it a new life? Wasn't it the same life transferred into a new body? So confusing.*

"That was easy, but I'm stuck wearing glasses for the rest of my life."

"It looks like it. Tsen said your severe astigmatism precludes contacts. Come on, wearing glasses isn't the end of the world. I've had mine since I was ten years old." Lishan showed him her satchel with his laptop and their game of Go. She also carried a recent copy of JAMA, featuring an article on the current status of tránsplants. "I stole this out of the library for you," she admitted, "so I'll have to take it back when you finish reading it. And I brought the Go, so tonight we might have something to do."

Lishan was sitting on the edge of his bed, where he reclined on his pillows. He pulled her down next to him. "I can think of several things we might do tonight that are better than playing Go." He kissed her passionately, and she participated fully, then stroked his groin.

"I love you. Get into bed with me, please."

"Slow down. I don't think this is the—" Lishan cautioned, but he stopped her with a kiss on the mouth. They both felt the swelling of his erection, signaling his readiness for the kind of intimacy they had never experienced with each other. They hungrily stroked one another and kissed every bit of exposed skin.

Suddenly, Lishan moved away. "Dear heart, we just can't do this now," she said breathlessly. "Someone might come into this room at any minute."

"No one will come in."

"There's no lock on the door."

"So what? I won't be embarrassed," he said.

"Well, I would. It has to be the right time and place. I want it as much as you, but I don't want our first time to be interrupted. I'm also on duty and have patients to see. Let's wait until we can make it as perfect as we can." They held hands for a long moment. Zicheng nodded, kissed her softly, and she slowly stood up and then backed out the door with a wave.

Within three days, Wong discharged Zicheng to return to the cottage. As Lishan helped pack his possessions, she said, "Ke, Sung, and your cook, Fong, will be glad to see you back. Sung has texted me almost every day since your surgery. He and Ke are going through the investigation and preparation for their transplants, so they're anxious to see how you have fared. Fong is planning to cook a special feast in your honor."

"I hope my taste sense returns by then. I remember Fong's attempt to replicate an American Thanksgiving dinner. In those days, I felt more like a biology specimen than a patient, but Fong fussed over us as though we were family." Another small piece fell into the puzzle.

Zicheng was beginning to recall living for several months with the other two candidates for surgery. The three men had become close friends, united by a bond of severe disability and the courage to try an unproven therapy. He was anxious to confirm his memories of these friends. He wondered about Lishan, who had mentioned living in the cottage and sleeping with him when he had no sex organs.

As she gathered his papers, he looked at her and said, "You're coming with me, aren't you?" She looked about to cry, then nodded several times and gave him a hug and three long kisses.

CHAPTER 5

Zicheng's return was a cottage celebration. Ke, Sung, and Fong welcomed Zicheng back with handshakes and laughter. Zicheng recognized the familiar smell, the light from the windows, his fellow patients, and the chubby cook, Fong.

"You've grown a full meter taller," joked Sung.

"You're a handsome Uyghur," added Ke. This remark puzzled Zicheng.

"Welcome back, Zicheng. Ignore those fools; they're just jealous," said Fong.

"Fong is correct," said Ke, looking sheepish. "We're happy with your result but impatient with our situation. They say that they'll do us soon, now that you have been such a big success. You make us very hopeful."

With some ceremony, Lishan appeared from the bedroom, driving the chariot. "Zicheng, say goodbye to your chariot. It now goes into honorable retirement. I'll run it over to physio."

"Wait a moment. I want to take a close look. It does bring back a lot of memories. I used it for about four months?"

"Yes, a few weeks in Chengdu and then over three months here in Harbin."

"I'll get my phone, so I can take a picture of you driving your creation." He took four shots to capture the image from all directions.

A new piece clicked into the recall jigsaw puzzle as the sight of the chariot brought back many memories, including the vision of Lishan in his bed.

"Thank you, Lishan, for designing and building it for me. I hope they never have another person like I was."

When Ke asked about his new mobility, Zicheng shuffled a few feet, pretending to do a little dance. As Lishan was returning the chariot, Fong produced a round of beers to grins all around.

"To Zicheng, welcome home," toasted Sung.

Fong announced to the smiling group that he would prepare "special lungs in milk soup and a delicious Dezhou braised chicken" for dinner.

When Zicheng heard the menu, he laughed, imagining that lungs would never make it onto his parents' menu at their Boston restaurant. Dinner conversation was in a mixture of Mandarin and English. Zicheng was pleased to find he understood most of the Mandarin phrases. The months of language tutoring before the transplant were now paying off.

At dinner, Zicheng forced himself to stay awake. Raising his wine glass, he said, "To Ke and Sung, may you get your operations soon and enjoy the same success I am having!"

By the time the dessert pastries were disappearing, the ever-protective Lishan, watching Zicheng fade, interrupted the chatter by rising from her chair. "Okay, I think Zicheng needs to go to bed! Say goodnight, Zicheng."

They walked into the bedroom, shut the door, and realized this would be the first time they would sleep together since the operation. Zicheng drew her into his arms in a tight hug. They kissed several times before Lishan suggested they should get ready for bed. She appeared tense, blushed slightly, and averted her gaze as he undressed. From a drawer, she drew out a long shirt that formerly was his daily garb. She held it out to him. "Do you mind?" she asked. He put it on as she went into the bathroom and emerged in her simple blue shift.

They lay down together, face to face, and suddenly embarrassment dissolved. Zicheng put one arm over her and looked steadily into her eyes. "As my memory returns, I realize that you've been my rock. I'm in love with a wonderful woman."

Lishan's heart quickened. "I think I love you, too," she replied, emphasizing the word "think." They both laughed as they linked their legs.

Gently rubbing her thigh, Zicheng said, "When we slept together before the operation, there was no possibility of sex. Now that I have a whole body, the possibility's there. But I'm so tired and so inept at controlling this new person that I'm not sure if my willing mind can get this body to pay attention."

Lishan kissed him on the mouth. He groaned. "Let's just take it as it comes," she said. "Excuse the poor pun." They grinned at each other, enjoying the warmth of their closeness. "Now relax," she said. She pulled back the sheet, moved her head down to his groin, and gave him the pleasure he had not experienced in months. He climaxed within a few minutes.

"Oh, my God. That was so wonderful. Thank you, thank you."

She pulled up the sheet and put her head on the pillow. They kissed again and fell asleep. Over the next few days, Zicheng found comfort in the now-familiar surroundings but was still fatigued by late afternoon. Then, one evening, a naked and smiling Lishan climbed into bed with him. The familiar warmth of her body, her kisses, and her exploring hands quickly banished his dark mood. She handed him a condom she had stowed under the pillow. "See if this fits," she said with a smile.

Zicheng quivered and knew without a doubt that his mind and body were in sync. The linking of a man and woman had never occurred with more emotion or enthusiasm. Zicheng lay silent in a warm glow. *I'm a real man again.*

The day after his return to the cottage, Zicheng had initiated a more vigorous exercise program. A Tai Chi class available on a television channel started every morning's activity. After breakfast, the occupational therapist supervised a set of movements. The hospital delivered an elliptical trainer, on which he spent an hour each day. Every afternoon, he took a long walk on the hospital grounds, although poor air quality took away any pleasure from the exercise.

An excited Sung was cutting open a box. "It finally came. I asked my boss to send me a virtual reality set and two programs I wrote. You should try one of these, Zicheng."

"That's what they call VR? I've heard of it but never tried such a thing."

"Did you ever play squash?" Sung asked.

"Oh, yeah. I played in high school and a bit in college, but I was never any good."

Sung gave him a brief tutorial, and within minutes, within a VR headset, Zicheng was swinging an imaginary racket.

Sung tapped Zicheng's shoulder. "Slow down, Zicheng, before you kill one of us. Try it outside."

He took full advantage of both of Sung's Virtual Reality programs that involved exercise. Within two weeks of returning to the cottage, his strength had markedly improved. Zicheng rediscovered the mirror.

In the privacy of his bedroom, he viewed his naked body. *Getting buffed. Actually, a handsome dude.*

One night, Zicheng asked his companions, "Is there ice skating here in Harbin?" Both men shrugged.

Fong overheard the question and replied, "You want speed skating, figure skating, ice dancing, hockey, or just skating? We have all of them indoors and outdoors. Harbin is a world center for winter sports. Indoor is better because our air quality is so poor."

Zicheng asked Lishan if she would like to go skating. She shook her head vigorously, "No way, I tried it once and kept falling. I'll watch you if you like." He suddenly realized that he would need to learn to skate all over again. That thought and Lishan's reaction shelved for the moment the idea of skating.

Talk of skating prodded Lishan. "Why don't we take in the Harbin Snow and Ice Festival? It's world famous, and I've never seen it."

"Sounds fine to me. I'm not sure I have the cold weather clothing for that kind of thing. Why don't we go shopping tomorrow and get proper gear?"

"I always enjoy shopping. It's a deal."

The next day at the mall, Zicheng was impressed by the variety of cold weather outerwear. Lishan gave a puzzled frown when Zicheng announced that it was better than the old Filene's basement. She selected a cashmere sweater, new boots, and a fur-trimmed anorak. Zicheng opted for a heavy-duty ski jacket with hood and ski pants. A knitted cap, fleece-lined high boots, sweater, gloves, and scarf completed his purchases. Lishan was pleasantly surprised that Zicheng insisted on paying for all of her items.

"Lishan, don't worry about it. Remember that I have an income, and you don't. I can afford it, and it gives me pleasure to buy you things." His American disability insurer had been quick to grant him his full benefits when he had sent them Lishan's picture of him post-hemicorporectomy in Chengdu. His income now exceeded that of most Chinese surgeons.

That Sunday, they took a taxi to the Snow and Ice Festival. Despite the bitter cold, they spent hours outdoors viewing the ice sculptures, several multicolored giant ice castles, and competitions that included ice-swimming. Like almost everyone there, they wore masks to protect against both the cold and foul air. They found a warm Chinese barbecue restaurant where they waited for the evening entertainment that included a spectacular fireworks display.

Zicheng commented, "I would never have imagined anything like this in China. I guess it makes sense that you make something out of it if you have a harsh and cold climate. Just like the Quebec City winter festival is famous for its ice sculptures and structures. Even Boston has a winter festival. I'm not sure I'm ready to stay in an ice hotel like they do in some Scandinavian countries. Of course, if you were there to keep me warm, it might be fun."

Lishan frowned. "Not my idea of fun, I mean, this has been a great day, but I'm not sure it would make me want to live in such a cold and awful place. Do you know that Harbin even has an indoor ski resort?"

Zicheng's head jerked up. "Indoor ski resort? You're kidding."

"I read it's the world's largest."

"I'll have to learn to ski all over again. Maybe next year, I'll be up to it."

Over the next few weeks, Zicheng's physical health continued to improve. However, by evening, he would be moody and irritable. He snapped at Fong and was unresponsive to Lishan's sexual advances. Almost every night, he dreamed of Joanne and would awake confused. His dreams brought memories of their courtship, their wedding, and her laugh. He could not discuss it with Lishan, who stiffened every time he mentioned Joanne. Zicheng realized that his mental status was far from satisfactory. Lishan expressed her concern about his mood swings when he became withdrawn and uncommunicative. After a few of these episodes, she spoke up, "I don't like the depressive moods you get. Were you like that in your life before the operation?"

"No, never,"

"Then why don't you go see Dr. Bin, the psychiatrist? Before your surgery, you seemed to get along well with him."

With luck, he was able to see Dr. Bin the following day. After hearing Zicheng's story, including the dreams about Joanne, Bin said, "You have been through a long and trying ordeal; you're now only six weeks post-op from that incredible operation. It seems as if most of your physical problems are behind you. Getting depressed after surgery or any major trauma is a common occurrence. I suggest a mild antidepressant for two or three months. We'll try a low dose of Paxil. How are you dealing with your body image?"

"It's getting much better, but I still have an occasional problem with some mirrors. My face doesn't look strange anymore. The dreams are more bothersome. Always about Joanne."

"Next visit, why don't you start from the beginning about your relationship with Joanne? Before your surgery, you gave me a quick summary, but it would help if we spent a little more time together. Take the pills until we meet again for a longer appointment. If the depression worsens, or you start thinking of suicide, call me right away. Will you promise?"

"I promise," Zicheng replied and booked an appointment for three weeks later.

CHAPTER 6

At the next Bin appointment, Zicheng described meeting Joanne during residency and the immediate attraction.

"And when did the sex begin?" Bin asked.

With a wry smile, Zicheng recounted their first sexual encounter. "We were in my apartment. I'm sitting on a soft leather hassock I had rescued from my parents' garage. Trying to balance, I swayed from side to side. Joanne is sitting astride my knees, kissing me and contributing to the rolling. When she pushed her chest against me, I feared I would fall backward.

"Whoa, you're going to cause an accident. We'll be the talk of the ER triage team when we explain our injuries."

"Scaredy cat. I thought this would be fun."

"I'm the one who'll get a skull fracture. I suggest bed, floor, or couch." His memory of their first sex was vivid. He had loved her playful sense of humor, the laughter in her speech, and the scent of her body.

They moved in together for the last six months of training. When they looked at job opportunities, since they were planning to marry, they sought positions in the same city. Denver had openings for both of them. They were excited to move west, near mountains and attractive job opportunities. They flew out for interviews. Two days later, Roger accepted a position at Denver General in the Emergency Department; Joanne would join a group practice in primary care. They married the week after their residencies finished. A motor trip to Denver was their honeymoon.

They elected to live a frugal lifestyle, pay off their student debts, and save for a down payment on a house. They waited a year before deciding to start a family.

Bin asked, "Were these decisions difficult?"

"Not really. We had no differences of opinion concerning family plans." At this point in his recitation, Zicheng felt he was narrating a movie. He recalled every detail of the worst year of his life.

After working several shifts at the hospital over the Labor Day holiday, Roger was glad to head home. Aware of Roger's schedule, Joanne had volunteered to be on-call for her practice, so her colleagues with children could enjoy the holiday weekend. They would have a simple dinner of steak and salad tonight, and tomorrow take a leisurely hike in the foothills, now empty of the weekend crowds. Hiking in the mountains was a reason they had chosen to live in Denver.

"And how is my mother-to-be tonight?" he asked, with a tired smile, a hug, and a kiss.

"Glad to finally be off-call, and I'm not a mother until next April, remember," referring to her first, and welcome, pregnancy. "No nausea the past three days, so the worst is over, I guess. I made your Manhattan and wish I could join you."

"I thought one drink was allowed."

"I know, but I'm doing this my way. No alcohol during pregnancy. I'll start the steaks while you have your drink."

After dinner on their condo patio, Joanne asked, "Would you look at my throat? It's been sore all weekend."

"Hey, I'm not your doctor. I should send you to the ER," he laughed as he walked toward her with his penlight and a kitchen spoon. Using the spoon handle as a tongue depressor, he peered down her throat, then felt under her chin. "It's only a little red, but your glands seem swollen. Tomorrow we'll stop by your office to get a swab done before we go on our walk."

At 8:30 the next morning, Joanne and Roger went to her office. To John Aiken, the first colleague she encountered in the hall, she said, "Roger thinks you should look at my throat and do a swab. Do you mind?"

Dr. Aiken examined her throat and then, as Roger had done earlier, felt around her neck for the lymph nodes and asked, "When did this start?"

"Probably about four days ago. It didn't bother me until yesterday. I thought it was just another of the viruses my patients bring me every day."

"You're probably right, so we'll do a throat swab before we start antibiotics. But while you're here, let's get a white count and mono test."

"You think I might have mononucleosis?"

"We'll see. I'll call you this afternoon when the labs are back."

"OK, thanks. Call my cell because we're going for a long hike."

The physician's assistant swabbed her throat and drew two vials of blood.

Roger drove the Jeep the hour to Summit Lake, one of their favorite places. On the uphill walk from the parking area, Joanne lagged; twice Roger helped her up a slope. "Hey, motherhood is slowing you down," he joked.

"Let me catch my breath. I feel my lack of exercise these last few months."

After an hour on the trail, seeing her grimaces and labored breathing, Roger said, "Let's cut it short, sit down, and eat our sandwiches. Then we'll head back." He tried to hide his concern.

"I'm out of shape; must be because I stopped my morning runs when the nausea started."

Roger nodded, "Maybe we should buy an elliptical trainer. I'd feel better about you using that rather than running on the streets. And, besides, I could use it myself."

"Good idea. Let's do that."

They finished the easy descent to the parking lot. On the drive back to Denver, Joanne's phone dinged a text message from her office, asking her to return to see Dr. Aiken before he left at 6 o'clock. She frowned, "Aiken wants to see me this afternoon. Should I be worried?" Roger shrugged and raised his eyebrows. Yes, he was worried.

Dr. Aiken saw them within minutes of their arrival. With a solemn face, he announced, "This doesn't look good. Your white count is 84,000, with a lot of immature white cells. You're a doctor, so you know that the most likely diagnosis at this time is leukemia. When I saw the lab results, I took the liberty of calling Ellen Gibbs' office. You know her. She's the best hematologist around. She's not in today, but her office gave you an appointment tomorrow morning at 8:30. I've faxed your lab work to her. I wish I had better news."

Joanne and Roger had both turned pale. Roger put his arm around her as she fought back her tears. "Did you know I'm pregnant?" she asked Aiken.

"No, but it makes your appointment tomorrow morning all the more important."

Roger supported Joanne as they said goodbye to Aiken and made their way to the Jeep. As he opened the car door, she broke into sobs.

He hugged her close, trying to reassure her. "We'll get through this, honey, we will." He helped her into the car. The drive home was silent except for Joanne's muffled sobs.

Roger made his Manhattan and heated a frozen pizza. "I will have a glass of red wine tonight," Joanne said. Then, pensively, "What other diagnosis could it be?"

"We're out of our areas of expertise. Let's not agonize all night thinking of alternatives. We know there are other possibilities a lot less dangerous than leukemia. Let's be hopeful and hold the questions for Dr. Gibbs tomorrow."

Dr. Gibbs took a detailed but quick medical history, then performed a thorough physical examination. She explained, "I'm not making a diagnosis at this point. We'll need a marrow biopsy and more blood work. I'll review some slides today, and the stains will be done overnight. I'll have a better opinion late tomorrow morning. We can do the biopsy right now." She led Joanne to a treatment room. Within minutes, she had anesthetized the hip area and collected the biopsy through a large needle. "Sorry, that stung a little. I'd like to see you back here tomorrow at noon."

"But what do you think?" asked Roger, looking anguished.

"I won't speculate since we will have more answers tomorrow."

At noon the next day, Roger and Joanne sat in Dr. Gibbs' consulting room. From behind her desk, the doctor looked solemn. "I'm afraid I have bad news. The marrow biopsy confirmed acute myelogenous leukemia. You know that AML has a high mortality rate, but we have some pretty effective treatments. I suggest we start with a chemo infusion here this afternoon. Can you come back in two hours?"

Bin interrupted, "That must have been very upsetting."

Zicheng responded, "The worst hour of my life to that point."

At lunch, Joanne ordered soup, tasted it, and left the remainder untouched. Roger choked down his hamburger with a beer. With moist eyes, Joanne spoke first. "I assume that the chemo will end my pregnancy. Do you think I should postpone the chemo?"

"Good question, but you don't leave AML for six months without treatment. Let's ask Gibbs when we go back."

Back in her office, Gibbs was firm. "I understand your concern, but this is a nasty disease, and I doubt that your pregnancy would be successful. I know it's a tough decision, but I advise you to start the chemo today and accept the consequences. We need to treat your AML; cure is a possibility, then you can deal with motherhood later."

"It sounds like I don't have much choice. Let's start the chemo."

As they started the IV for the infusion, Gibbs continued her explanation concerning the course of treatment and the likelihood of a miscarriage. She added, "Take whatever you like for any nausea. It won't interfere with the treatment. Call me anytime you have a concern or questions." As she patted Joanne's hand, she said, "I know this is one of the worst days of your life. When you miscarry, come into the hospital where we can monitor your blood loss. Understand?"

Joanne nodded as she started to sob in silence. Roger held her hand.

Within a week of the first infusion, Joanne lost the pregnancy. Although she was in hospital overnight, blood loss was minimal. A weekly trip to Gibbs' office would sometimes include a chemo infusion, sometimes a blood transfusion for the next few months. She found the trips tiring and depressing. Roger was frustrated at his inability to help her.

By the second week of December, Roger doubted the efficacy of Joanne's treatment. He arranged a personal appointment with Dr. Gibbs.

"Joanne is not doing too well. What's next for her?"

"We have one more chemo drug I'd like to try. If that doesn't work, a marrow transplant is our only option left."

"Would you be hurt if I asked for a second opinion somewhere else?"

"I always favor second opinions. Where were you thinking about?"

"You know more about that than I do. What do you consider the centers of excellence?"

"Well, it's between Cedars-Sinai in Los Angeles or Dana-Farber in Boston."

"Boston's my hometown. If they're equivalent, I'd opt for Dana-Farber."

"I did my fellowship year there, so I know the people. I'll get her records organized and talk to Sam Stein. He's head of hematology; we're old friends. Give me a week to get back to you." Within a week, Dr. Gibbs had spoken to Stein at Dana-Farber, summarized the medical records, and sent him representative microscope slides from the bone marrow biopsy.

At Christmas, Joanne was still living at home with constant fatigue and chronic nausea. Her parents had retired and moved to Denver to be near her during her illness.

On New Year's Day, Joanne entered the kitchen and found Roger staring out their kitchen window, a cup of coffee growing cold on the counter. "Rog," Joanne said, "we're going skating today."

"Are you sure? I don't think you're up to it."

"We've done it every year for the past five years, with or without hangovers."

"Whatever you say, dear," Roger shrugged.

She wore a knitted cap to cover her bald head. They were at a large outdoor skating rink an hour later, under brilliant blue skies with music blaring. On the ice, children chased one another like swarms of flies. A young woman in a figure skating costume looked out of place as she practiced jumps and spins. Two couples in their twenties glided together around the oval. A few middle-aged women, their faces tense, shuffled around the margins, gripping the boards.

Joanne sat on a bench as Roger laced up her white figure skates. After he donned his battered hockey skates, they took off together, Roger linking their right hands with his left arm around her waist. Nearly halfway around the rink, she suddenly clutched his arm and started to collapse. In one quick motion, he grabbed her waist, lifted her, and carried her back to the bench at the rink-side. As he unlaced and removed her skates, Joanne whispered, "I'm sorry, take me home," and dabbed at her eyes with a tissue.

"Don't worry about it, hon. You tried."

Back home, Joanne was solemn. "We have to talk. The treatment isn't working. I'm going to die. My quality-of-life sucks. I'm not doing any more chemo."

"Wait a minute. We don't give up that quickly. For the past few weeks, I've been thinking about an alternative. I'm not happy with your lack of progress. Let's go back to Boston for another opinion. The Dana-Farber Institute is the best in the world."

"I'm not up to the travel just to get another opinion."

"It's more than a second opinion. Gibbs and I have already talked to them and sent your records. They're interested in putting you into a trial they're running. I also checked out the travel. We can charter a business jet and get you there tomorrow."

"You didn't tell me anything about this plan."

"I was waiting until after the holiday, but I've been working on it for almost a month."

"Roger, you're always doing things like that without asking *me*. It'll cost a fortune. Don't waste our money on me."

"It's not that expensive. We have the money, and it's not a waste. I'm anxious to do this."

"Oh, Rog. Are you sure they have a different treatment?"

"They have several trials underway. Dr. Gibbs recommends this. Let's give it a chance."

"Would you come with me?"

"Of course. I'll never leave you on your own. I've even arranged coverage for me at the hospital. We can leave tomorrow if the flight is still available."

"I'll say yes, but help me to the bed. I have to lie down. And I need another pain pill."

When she settled in, Roger moved to the living room, and credit card in hand, he called the charter service. Yes, they had a flight available tomorrow morning. They would arrive in Boston at 4 pm. He then booked a hotel near Dana-Farber, sent an e-mail to his colleague replacing him while away, and called Joanne's parents, who arranged to see them off at the Denver airport.

He called his father and explained the arrangements for the Dana-Farber. His father would pick them up at the General Aviation terminal tomorrow.

Joanne sprawled out and slept most of the way on the business jet. At the Boston Marriot, exhausted by the trip, she declined dinner and fell asleep while Roger had room service. The next morning, Roger wheeled her to a taxi.

"Roger, if this doesn't work out, get me home to die. I want to die in *my* bed, not in a Boston hospital."

"You didn't come here to die. You're going to get the best treatment in the world."

Dr. Stein's staff attacked for four days, taking countless blood samples, another marrow biopsy, and doing CT, MRI, and PET scans.

Roger refused to stay at the hotel, insisting on sleeping on the couch in Joanne's room. He brought his food from the hospital cafeteria to her room.

"So where is the magic treatment, Roger? I feel like a science experiment. I want to know what's going on. It's my body; I have a say."

"I've asked for a conference with the team for this afternoon to see what happens next."

"Have the meeting here. I'm entitled to hear it all," Joanne said.

"Yes, honey. No one is holding anything back from you."

That afternoon, a grim-faced Dr. Stein, his teaching fellow at his side, faced Roger and Joanne. "Not good news, I'm afraid. Joanne, you're not going into one of our trials. We found you have a fungal infection in your lungs and blood. You know that's a common complication of chemotherapy. Right now, we have no treatment for that particular strain. We're looking around the world to see if anyone has an antifungal drug we don't have."

Roger spoke up, "I know that you oncologists have an international network. How long before you have any answers?"

Joanne interrupted. "Roger, cut the crap! They aren't going to treat me. Get that damn plane back, and get me home. I'll die in my own bed with you and my parents around. Let's go *now.*"

Dr. Stein looked uncomfortable and nodded slightly.

"Okay, dear," Roger whispered. "I'll get you home as soon as I can."

The next day, Roger carried her bald and pale form from the business jet to the waiting Denver ambulance. At home in her bed, Joanne tried to comfort him. "Roger, don't be so hard on yourself. You did everything to make it work, but sometimes you must give up. I'm ready to die; you have to be ready for it."

"I have a problem with that." His chin was trembling.

"Make sure I get enough pain meds. You can do that. And when I'm gone, get back to your career and find another wife. You deserve the children you and I never had. Promise me that."

His dry mouth made his response almost inaudible. "I can't even think about that."

That night, about 3 a.m., Joanne suddenly coughed a large amount of bright blood and fell back, unconscious, waking Roger. He sat upright, felt for a pulse in her neck, and started to weep.

"A very difficult experience," Bin commented. "Your story helps me understand some of your problems."

Roger buried Joanne in a shroud, her pine forest grave unmarked as she had directed him. The small crowd of mourners included Roger's and Joanne's parents, her sister Charlene, and a dozen Denver friends. They all attended the memorial service later that week in their local Unitarian Universalist Church.

He missed Joanne's company at meals; her absence from his bed left him sleepless. He declined several dinner invitations—he was not yet ready to socialize. With his usual determination, he plunged himself into his work, taking on many extra hours. He did evening shifts at a charity clinic for the homeless. After a month of an exhausting schedule, he took three days hiking alone on Mt. Evans to clear his head.

Will Willoughby, his closest medical colleague, took him aside, "Roger, I won't ask you how it's going. You look like shit. What can I do for you?"

"It's tough. No matter how much I should have anticipated Joanne's death, it didn't help. Nothing prepares you for this. If I were more depressed, I'd see a shrink and get some antidepressants, but I'm not there yet. Working extra keeps my mind busy, but I'm still going to have to face the future. I'm wondering about taking some time off."

"That might be a good idea. But I think you need some Prozac or Zoloft or something."

Later that week, Roger stopped a psychiatrist colleague at the hospital, took him aside, and explained his situation. The "curbside consult" resulted in a Zoloft prescription with no refills and an admonition for Roger to make an office visit next time. When Roger got home that night, he recalled the Tibet trip he and Joanne had planned.

Before her pregnancy, Joanne had prepared a folder of information for Tibet. When he reviewed it, he realized that some of the information was probably out of date. Over the next two weeks, Roger confirmed the availability of the guided trek. He ascertained visa requirements and available airline connections. In updating her research, he was concerned by what he read about China-Tibet issues and the Dalai Lama conflict. He had considerable correspondence with the guiding firm before buying the trip.

Bin said, "So that explains how you got to Tibet before the accident. I had wondered about that."

CHAPTER 7

"Zicheng, in Chengdu, you had retrograde amnesia from the concussion in Tibet. It's not important. It was a good thing for you to review your life with Joanne. I see that you were a loving and compassionate husband. I suggest we talk next time about your time in the hospital in Chengdu. You have a clear case of PTSD; we need to help you with that."

Zicheng was shocked at Bin's diagnosis of PTSD. Still, Bin was confident. "Zicheng, it's obvious. In one year, you have had several traumatic experiences. Losing a spouse is always considered one of the most dangerous threats to your mental health. And then you lost half your body in a car accident. Then after that, you had one of the most incredible surgical operations ever completed."

"I never thought of PTSD, even though it was common enough in the ER patients. So, what's the treatment?"

"First, you need to accept the diagnosis. Then I suggest you tell Lishan for her to understand you better. Continue taking Paxil. Don't mix it with booze; that's dangerous, and you know it. You should do some reading on PTSD to understand yourself a little better. It's a chronic disease. Don't expect it to disappear next week. I'd like to see you in two weeks after the Paxil has had more time to work. If you get more depressed or suicidal, you call me immediately at any hour. Understand?"

Zicheng accepted the prescription and booked his return appointment as he left to walk back to the apartment. He felt frustrated that he had not thought of the diagnosis. He faced Lishan when she arrived home just before midnight.

"Lishan, we have to talk about something important."

"Right now? I'm so tired I can hardly think."

"It's about me. I have PTSD. Peter Bin says so."

"You saw him today? I didn't know you were going."

"We spent over an hour. Bin thinks it's pretty clear."

She embraced him. "Whatever can I do to help?"

"Just understand and forgive me for being less of a partner for you. I've been preoccupied with my problems and not listening to yours."

"We'll get through this. I'm glad you told me, though. But let's talk about it more when I'm in better shape. I'm back on duty in six hours."

"I understand. Thank you for understanding. Now get to bed."

For the next week, Lishan made daily inquiries of Zicheng concerning his health and reassured him she was there to help in any way. The Paxil gradually decreased the Joanne nightmares, and that issue subsided. As he improved, Zicheng reflected on the magnitude of his experience, the near-miraculous surgery, and the extent of his recovery. He was grateful for the care in Chengdu and Harbin.

Meanwhile, the recurrent testing, blood draws, x-rays, and urinalyses continued to annoy him. At his next meeting at the Institute, Wong gave him the results of his recent psychometric testing, showing an IQ of 132 and good functioning on all other parameters. Zicheng now had normal blood results and good kidney function.

"Why do I need yet another eye exam?"

Dr. Wong asked, "Do you remember your pre-op eye and hearing exams?"

"I'm afraid I still have a lot of gaps in my memory, especially events between Chengdu and my surgery."

"We did visual field testing. We want to repeat that to see if the operation damaged your vision. Our concern is more to document our research results than any thought that you would need treatment. The test will take about an hour."

"But I had an eye exam since the surgery. That's when I got my glasses."

In his usual flat monotone and with no facial expression, Wong shrugged and replied, "They didn't do your visual fields in that exam. We want your data to be complete."

Once again, Zicheng felt irritated at being treated like a biology specimen.

His steady work on the elliptical trainer and regular strength-training exercise now showed results. When he mentioned his desire to soon return to some kind of work, Wong suggested, "Would you like to work here in the animal surgery lab? It would give you a chance to see if you can regain your surgical skills."

"Are you serious? I would be delighted. When do I start?"

Wong answered, "Li and I've been discussing this for some time. There's no pay. Li will be your supervisor. Consider it an apprenticeship."

"Can I start tomorrow?"

"Be at the animal lab at eight o'clock. Li will show you what to do."

"Thank you. You and the rest of the staff saved my life; now you are giving me the hope of a future."

Zicheng returned to the cottage in good spirits; he was firmly back on the road to recovery. He took Lishan to dinner that evening. Despite sleeping together since returning to the cottage, Zicheng and Lishan had little awake time together due to her hospital schedule. When they were together, he had shown little interest in sex for weeks.

"Lishan, look how far I've come. Tomorrow I start work at the lab. It's not the practice of medicine but a far cry from when I was Roger in Chengdu."

"I'm very proud of you. I don't think I've ever seen anyone work harder. You deserve every success. Here's to you!" She raised her glass.

"Here's to us. You're the one who got me through some tough times."

"Let's have a proper graduation test. Fong always gives you a knife and fork. It's time you graduated to chopsticks."

"You must be kidding."

Lishan removed his fork from his plate and handed him the chopsticks. He first contorted his face, then broke into a smile as he tried to grip the unfamiliar tools.

"Look, hold them like this," as she put her hand and sticks next to his. "And get the length right. Too far up or down, and you lose either control or pressure on the food."

To the surprise of them both, Zicheng quickly mastered picking up morsels of pork and carrots. As he viewed the rice bowl with suspicion, Lishan spoke up, "If you've watched me all this time, you will have noticed that I pick up the bowl and put it right under my mouth. You will do the same with *fun*, you know, the noodles." With some skepticism and occasional sprays of rice onto the tabletop, he began to feel more comfortable with his new utensils. After several more mouthfuls, he decided to complete the dinner *sans fork*.

Over dinner, they discussed their plans since Zicheng would have to stay at least another six months in Harbin to continue the lower dose of Dr. Chu's antirejection drug. Lishan would graduate from medical school in early May. They planned for her months' vacation before residency training. They would travel around China. She would take him to her home village; he would introduce her to camping and hiking, although she showed little enthusiasm for sleeping in a tent. In bed that night, their prospects propelled them into a noisier-than-usual passion. The morning after, Zicheng concluded that his relationship with Lishan was recovering; the future was brighter.

CHAPTER 8

Walking to the animal lab wearing hospital scrubs gave Zicheng a feeling of optimism and excitement, mixed with anxiety over his need to succeed. He knew that he now had an opportunity for full rehabilitation. His recent mastery of chopsticks boosted his confidence that he would be able to handle surgical instruments.

Zicheng's rhythmic footsteps to the lab reactivated the earworm, present since the week after his Chengdu hemicorporectomy, when he first saw his shortened body. The words were from an Irish folk song his father sometimes sang after boisterous family holiday meals.

Where are the legs with which you run
When you first went to carry a gun
Indeed your dancing days are done
Oh Johnny, I hardly knew ye....
Ye're an armless, boneless, chickenless egg
Ye'll have to be put in a barrel to beg
Oh Johnny, I hardly knew ye.

Li met him just inside the doorway and shook his hand. "Welcome to the Institute surgical team. Maybe we'll make you a veterinary surgeon by practicing on animals. We're lucky we have no restrictions on the use of animals, so we can perfect our surgical techniques and do transplant experiments." Zicheng recoiled, realizing that this practice would not happen in an American institution unless approved by an animal care committee.

When they entered the large animal area, a definite barnyard smell hit their nostrils. Immediately, they saw two pens, each holding four spotted pigs. After passing those, a group of six gorillas in a room-size cage noisily heralded their arrival.

Passing that cage, Li unlocked a smaller door through which he led Zicheng. Now they saw two gorillas similar to the previous lot. In this room, however, each animal lived in a separate space. Gorilla number one was eating a banana, while gorilla number two leaned against a wall, snoring. After a whistle from Li, they both came to attention and stared at the visitors. "Here you see one of our experiments from about ten months ago. These are twins, and in one operation, we exchanged their brains. In earlier experiments, we swapped whole heads. It worked, but there were problems with the pharyngeal structures that control swallowing. We decided to, in the future, move brains instead of heads. It means more work dealing with the cranial nerves, but it's working.

As you can see, they have survived well. Both animals still have some vision problems, but they move well and communicate with each other. We have not made this experiment public at this time, so please observe our confidentiality rules, just as you protect your privacy."

In a small conference room, Li explained their progress. "We are happy with the success with the two gorillas," he began, "because we have demonstrated the feasibility of connecting the vascular and nervous systems in these animals. Because they are identical twins, we have not had any severe rejection phenomenon, although we watch them closely, and we're prepared to treat any such reactions.

"Two months after the gorilla operation, we performed a similar procedure on two human volunteers. Since we had no twins available, we were more concerned about rejection issues. We stored a large marrow sample from each. We used radiation and chemotherapy to obliterate any marrow remaining in their bones. We then replaced the marrow in each with that from the other volunteer. That meant that each of them was living with a donor blood and immune system. After about 100 days, we exchanged brains in the same fashion as with the gorillas. Both men survived a full six months, and we followed their sensory and motor functions closely. We consider the operation to be a success, but we must be cautious in our optimism."

"And what happened to the men?"

"Unfortunately, under our agreement with the authorities, we had to sacrifice the prisoners six months after the transplants."

"Sacrifice? You mean you killed them?"

"We had no choice. They were prisoners that always understood they would be given lethal injections at the end of the experiment. When they volunteered, they knew the agreement. The prisoners each gained about a year of life by participating. They considered it fair and gave informed consent."

"And you consider your surgery was ethical?"

"Absolutely, but we won't need to do any more healthy volunteers. We now have patients like you. Come along here and see something interesting. Welcome to our pathology museum." He opened an unmarked door. On shelves around the room were various organs, sealed in clear plastic boxes and floating in formaldehyde. Zicheng remembered studying such displays as a medical student.

"Many of these are specimens from previous animal experiments.

You can read the story of each specimen on the card below. But let me show you one that's not a real organ specimen."

He pulled out a larger container. A white plastic skull, top removed at the brow line, rested in the box. Within the cranial cavity glistened a pinkish brain covered by its arachnoid membrane. A white tag identified each nerve, a red tag was on each artery, and a blue tag on every vein. "Zicheng, you're now looking at a perfect model of your brain."

"What?" He leaned forward, examining the ridges and valleys of his cerebral cortex.

"You remember when I took you to the radiology department a few days before your surgery?"

"Oh vaguely, x-rays, CT scan, and MRI. The works."

"From those images, we programmed a 3-D printer to make a replica of your brain out of a jelly-like substance."

"It's amazing. Even the color looks like a living brain."

"Our medical artist matched the colors when she programmed the printer. But get this: when she did it, she made three brains; Wong and I used two of her models to rehearse your surgery. To make the skull, we imaged the donor and printed a copy of his skull. We checked the fit of your brain into his skull. We saw what we would need to connect all the nerves and blood vessels. When we finished the connections and were ready to close at your operation, we placed several microsensors on your brain surface to transmit signals of the brain activity through the skull. It creates an EEG that is more accurate than conventional EEGs taken outside the skull."

"Stunning," Zicheng whispered. "I'm looking at my brain." He shivered. *Wait till I tell Lishan about this.* During his recovery in the hospital room, he had noticed the EEG machine but was unaware he had intracranial sensors transmitting his EEG.

"I thought you would like that. Let's finish the tour." They continued along the hallway.

"So, you have two fully-equipped operating rooms, each with a robotic operating microscope and two smaller ORs?"

"Yeah, we use the smaller ones for most animals, and we use the larger rooms for primates. When we did the human experiment, we used the hospital OR. We use the same sterile surgical techniques on animals as we do on humans. We're developing procedures that we can replicate on patients. The impressive thing to me is the goal of performing human brain transplants. The devil is always in the details—joining nerves, arteries, and veins. To perfect our technique, we do other things. This morning, we have scheduled a kidney transplant into a pig. Perhaps you'd like to scrub in as an assistant while I do the actual transplant."

"I love that idea. This is a big opportunity for me." He had a sudden flutter in his pulse—this would be the first test of his surgical abilities since the transplant. He looked at his calloused and heavy laborer hands. He was missing the nail of his right index finger, a white scar in its place. Would he be able to control these thick and clumsy fingers?

They scrubbed using the proper technique at the sink and went into the OR to find an intubated unconscious pig lying on a gurney under bright lights. Two masked technicians were shaving and scrubbing the incision site before applying the usual drapes. During the surgery, Zicheng's role was confined mostly to holding retractors. Li removed the kidney, inserted the donor organ, connected the blood supply and ureter, then suggested, "I think you should close while I assist."

A ripple of excitement coursed through Zicheng's body. Holding the needle driver to suture the fascia and muscles felt strangely unfamiliar. His new fingers had no memory of doing a task he had formerly done many times. He concentrated on the chore.

"I'm slow and clumsy. Do you want to take over?"

"We have lots of time."

He finally had the muscles pulled together. As he expected, Li scrutinized his progress.

"Well done. I'll let you close on your own." He stepped away but continued watching.

Zicheng was anxious to finish the operation. Starting to close the skin, his hand shook slightly with the first staple.

"I'm not doing too well, Li."

"You're fine. Just take your time. You haven't been doing this for quite a while. I'm going to scrub out and leave you to it."

Zicheng was pleasantly surprised at Li placing such confidence in him. He felt like a surgeon again. With new confidence, he moved faster and did not shake on the second staple. He was into a rhythm by the third, then continued until he finished a straight staple line for a clean and even closure. Zicheng's sweat showed on his forehead as he stepped away from the table. "Thanks for letting me do that. I know I can get better," he said.

"That's why you're here," replied Li. "It's obvious you know what you're doing, but your technique may be a little, well, rusty." He smiled and gave a thumbs-up sign, indicating he could give Dr. Wong a promising report.

As he walked back to the cottage, Zicheng was pleased as he looked at his future. *I'll get better with some practice.* His pocket held a spool of 4-0 suture material, a needle driver, a Kelly clamp, and scissors. He would rehearse his technique on an orange at home.

That morning he had spoken not one word of English; Mandarin was his working language. Prior to his transplant, he had Mandarin lessons daily. He now met his tutor Lee Shang only once a week, and they concentrated more on pronunciation than vocabulary or grammar. Chinese characters were still a problem, but his reading was improving. He now understood many of the stories in the local newspaper.

He was anxious to see Lishan at dinner. He spoke almost non-stop through the meal, still excited at the day's events.

"This sounds like the best day since your transplant. I'm so happy for you."

"Don't forget, you helped me get to this place. I feel like today changed our lives."

Later, in bed that night, Lishan asked, "Every night, you stay up reading that damn Kindle. Why is it important?"

"To read the Globe. It's my hometown newspaper. I've been reading it since I was a kid. Even in Denver, I read the Globe."

"You should remember you're now Zicheng, not Roger. Good night." She turned over to sleep.

Zicheng told Ke and Sung that he was working in the laboratory. He did not mention doing surgery, and his housemates asked no questions about his duties. The success of Zicheng's transplant produced an atmosphere of optimism in the house. His two housemates and Fong were addicted to the Kung Fu programs on the television. In his previous life, Zicheng had never been interested in martial arts but was gaining an appreciation through his exposure almost every evening. Zicheng offered to take Fong and his housemates to an international Kung Fu tournament in Harbin. When Lishan declined to attend, the four men went together to the evening event. Zicheng was intrigued by the sport. The men enjoyed a few beers and many laughs, significantly when one of the fighters fell from the ring and platform into the audience. Zicheng realized that this was his first social outing in a group. He felt comfortable in the situation. His mastery of Mandarin allowed him to appreciate jokes and make witty comments.

The day after the tournament, Zicheng asked Dr. Wong, "I was watching some Kung Fu. Is there any reason I can't try martial arts?"

"You have almost no restrictions, but I would be concerned about a possible weakness at the base of your skull where we cut the spinal cord. I would not recommend martial arts. You told us you were doing Tai Chi. That is safe; I've done it every day for the past twenty years."

"Thank you. I'm disappointed but glad I asked first. I'll remain a spectator for the Kung Fu."

Back at the cottage, Ke took him aside. In a voice distorted by his old burn injuries, he said, "Zicheng, I cannot tell Sung, but they have scheduled me for the marrow extraction. That means I'll be next."

"Good news, Ke. I hope you do as well as me."

The next day, at the laboratory, Zicheng stopped Li in the corridor. "Ke tells me he has to give a marrow sample tomorrow to get ready for his surgery. What is that about?"

"Remember your experience. We knocked out the donor's marrow with drugs and radiation, then gave him a marrow transplant from you. We did that to reduce rejection. So you carry your original marrow and immune system. We explained it to you before surgery, but I guess your recall is still not quite complete."

Several more images snapped into Zicheng's memory.

During his first apprenticeship week, Zicheng helped the technicians with post-op care of the animals and assisted in one more transplant. The regular lab schedule included two or three operations per week. Li allowed Zicheng to use dead animals to practice surgical dissection, ligation (ties), and wound closure. He concentrated hard on each procedure—write out the steps, imagine the hand movements, assemble the tools, review the steps, and then perform the operation. His frustration with his clumsy fingers was sometimes overwhelming, and others in the lab got used to hearing his growls and curses. Each day he improved his skills and grew his confidence.

After four weeks of watching Zicheng improve, Li told Zicheng, "In two weeks, we're going to do a gorilla-to-gorilla hand transplant. Wong and I would like you to remove the donor animal hand and then help me do the attachment on the recipient. How does that sound?"

"I like that challenge! This afternoon I'll start reviewing my hand and wrist anatomy. Can I assume the gorilla structures are the same as in humans?'

"The structures are virtually identical, so you won't have any problems if you refresh your memory of the anatomy. We can have fun doing this together."

That afternoon in the medical library, Zicheng found the traditional Grey's Anatomy and a specialized textbook on hand and wrist anatomy. Over four evenings, he memorized the relationships. In the privacy of his bedroom, he continued to practice tying knots and suturing. He was confident that his brain was sending muscle-memory messages to his new hands. With time and his frequent scrubs, the heavy callouses were disappearing, along with the tobacco stains.

Lishan paid close attention to his surgical practice. "You're serious about this gorilla operation," she said.

"Of course. It's an opportunity for me but a challenge. I'm confident about the anatomy, but I worry I'll be clumsy in doing the surgery. I don't want to blow it in front of Wong and Li."

On May 2, Zicheng severed the hand of one gorilla while Li did the other, both under Wong's watchful eyes. The two surgeons then swapped stations, and Zicheng had the challenge of attaching his gorilla's hand to the other animal. The operation took five hours, with Li finishing only slightly before Zicheng.

Wong invited Zicheng to a restaurant lunch to celebrate the surgery. Raising his beer glass, Wong toasted his two proteges. "You were both excellent. Zicheng, I enjoyed watching your progress with the robotic microsurgery. You learn fast."

"It's a great privilege to have this training. I've learned so much in such a short time. Thank you both."

"We've another matter to discuss. What's the state of your tourist visa?"

Looking at his original U.S. Roger Scully passport and its visa page, Zicheng replied, "Oh-oh, my visa expired the first of March."

"That could be a problem. The hospital has a team of federal officials visiting for the next week. They're checking the documentation of all staff and patients."

"What should I do?"

"We have to get your status adjusted. Don't do anything on your own. I'll have our Beijing attorney deal with it. I'll call him today. In the meantime, don't leave the hospital grounds but stay in the cottage and lab building. Stay out of the main hospital complex. We don't want you deported."

Zicheng was concerned but skeptical at Wong's motives. *Does he want to help me or continue adding data to his study? If the authorities deport me back to the States, what will happen to my rejection drug treatment?*

CHAPTER 9

Wong's question about the visa gave Zicheng another concern— his passport. His photo did not resemble his face. Preoccupation with survival and recovery had caused him to neglect bureaucratic needs like passport and visa. He contacted Mr. Metcalf at the Chengdu consulate to discuss arrangements for a new passport. Metcalf was delighted to hear of Zicheng's progress since he had visited Zicheng (who he remembered as Roger Scully) in the Chengdu hospital.

"You have to be careful. With an expired visa and the wrong passport photo, the Chinese could immediately deport you. I'll make a call, and you should expect to hear from the Beijing embassy within 24 hours."

Sure enough, within four hours, Mr. Smothers, a Beijing undersecretary, called to set up an appointment. He told Zicheng to bring his current passport. He gave the name of a photographer's shop near the embassy, where Zicheng would be sure to get passport photos of biometric quality. They agreed on a date and time to meet the following week.

When he informed Wong of his appointment, Wong said, "I'm giving you the name and telephone number of Mr. Leung to meet in

Beijing while you are there. He's expecting to hear from you. He's very well-connected, and I am sure he can get your visa renewed or reissued. You might have a problem traveling by airline with your current documents. Therefore, Mr. Moon has kindly offered you the use of his plane that brought you here from Chengdu."

"Is this the man who has been paying all my bills and treating me so well?"

"You might meet him later. He is a man of great wealth, born in this country but living in Singapore. Mr. Moon has long funded this Institute, for which we are most grateful. However, he avoids publicity and doesn't want recognition for his contribution. He's been following your progress carefully and is delighted that his investment has shown such a good result. The lawyer you will meet in Beijing works for Mr. Moon." Later in the day, Leung messaged that they would meet with the Chinese officials immediately after Zicheng's passport renewal.

Zicheng was pleased he would soon solve the passport problem. Remembering Wong's warning, he was no longer confident to walk around downtown Harbin, making simple conversation in Mandarin. Away from the Institute and the hospital's sheltered environment, he felt vulnerable, like a chick from a new-hatched egg.

He discussed his fears with Lishan. "I have to keep a low profile until I get my passport and visa. I should've thought of it before. Once I have those things cleared, I'll feel more like a free man. A passport that doesn't match my face would be sure to land me in jail."

"You worry too much. Another week, and you'll have everything cleared up."

"With the new passport, I'll be able to fly home for a visit. And a new visa will get me back into China."

"If you go to America for a visit, I probably won't be able to travel with you. The way China-US relations are going, they probably wouldn't give me a visa. I'm worried you won't want to come back."

"Of course, I'll be back. I have you and my treatment here."

"I'm glad to hear that. I understand that you want to see your parents again, but I'll be glad to have you back with me."

Zicheng stood naked at the bedside. Lishan smiled and said, "You're a big improvement over the man I met in Chengdu."

"So, do you now see me as American or as Chinese?"

She raised her eyebrows, paused to purse her lips, then spoke. "What if I said neither?"

"Neither?" he gasped. "Neither Chinese nor American? I'm confused."

"Well, I don't want to upset you and worry about it, but your face and skin are more like a Uyghur than a regular Han Chinese. It doesn't matter to me, but you should understand that many Chinese do not recognize Uyghurs as Chinese. We're Han. They're Turks!"

His pulse rose. "I can't believe this. I think I'm Chinese, and you're telling me I'm a Turk? What am I?"

"Well, not exactly a Turk. Uyghurs come from Turkestan and have a different language. They cause a lot of trouble for our country."

"I had read a bit about it but didn't give it much thought. When I discovered I was circumcised, it briefly crossed my mind that the donor had been Muslim."

"Zicheng, don't worry about it. I think of you as Zicheng, not American, Chinese, or Uyghur."

An hour of intense passion initiated by Lishan obliterated his immediate identity concern. However, for the next few days, Zicheng reflected on the race issue. *I am who I am and shouldn't worry about looking like a Uyghur. I'm pretty handsome. Lishan's fine with my looks. I should ask her to marry me.*

He planned the occasion. He reserved a table at Ubugema, Harbin's most expensive restaurant. Lishan was surprised. "What's the big occasion? I thought you were staying out of public view."

"I'm sure no one will be checking IDs at the restaurant. We have things to discuss before I go to Beijing in two days."

After making their choices from the steakhouse menu, sitting next to Lishan, Zicheng raised his wine glass and asked, "Will you marry me? I want to spend our lives together."

"Wow, that's a pleasant surprise. I'd love to marry you. You know I love you, but we're still sorting out some problems. I'm flattered, and I like the idea; I was hoping you would ask me someday."

"What's the problem?"

"We have to be practical and see how you make out in Beijing. When your status is clear, then we'll discuss marriage. I want it to happen." She turned and kissed him, then moved closer along the banquette. He enjoyed the warmth of her body with the heady rose scent she was wearing.

"Let's assume it'll work out. Wong seemed confident that the lawyer and Mr. Moon will make everything happen. How are you going to deal with your family?"

"I need to think about that. It might be best to get my brother on my side first. We'll figure a way to change their minds."

The next day at the laboratory, Wong handed him a folder and said, "We now consider you more a member of our team than a patient. Here is the manuscript that Dr. Li and I prepared this week for submission to *Lancet*, describing your successful body transplant. As you will see, there is no mention of your name, race, or nationality. Until the paper is published, please treat it as highly confidential. You may share it only with your friend, Miss Zhou Lishan."

That evening, he and Lishan pored over the paper, written in English, and prepared for the prestigious journal. "Well, this will be a sensation in the medical world and the lay press. Wong and Li know they will receive a lot of attention, with everyone trying to discern my identity. I hope there are no leaks from the hospital or the Institute. I don't want that kind of publicity."

"You're right. Maybe the paper will come out when we're away on vacation. What will it be like for us when you become world famous?"

"I don't see myself as becoming famous. I'm just the subject of a surgical experiment."

"You underestimate your importance."

The flight to Beijing on Mr. Moon's plane took an hour and 15 minutes; he took a taxi to the St. Regis hotel, where the embassy had pre-registered Roger Scully to avoid the need for him to show documentation. He deposited his backpack in his room and made his way down to the bar, where he enjoyed a Manhattan before having an excellent dinner in the dining room. The touristy Peking duck dinner was a welcome change from Fong's stews.

Back in his room, he called Lishan to announce his safe arrival. They both knew the importance of tomorrow's appointment.

In the morning, he took a taxi to the photography shop recommended by the embassy. Within 20 minutes, he had the necessary pictures. A nervous Roger walked to the U.S. Embassy. The receptionist checked her computer screen and placed a call, then said that someone would come and escort him. He barely had time to step aside when a distinguished-looking white gentleman appeared. "Good morning, doctor. I'm Leonard Smothers. We've been expecting you, and this will only take a few minutes if you just follow me."

They passed a security guard and entered a door labeled "Passport Section." Smothers looked at the photographs, approved them, and gave Roger a simple form to complete. He did not comment on the change in appearance since the issuance of the previous passport. "Are you paying by credit card?" asked Smothers. *I guess I'm going to get the passport.* Roger handed him the American Visa card. "It will take about two hours to prepare your passport, so it should be ready by lunchtime. It'll be waiting for you at the front desk. I suggest you get a new visa as soon as possible." He returned the Visa card and old passport. "Is there anything else I can do for you?"

"No, thank you," Roger said. "I'm pleased to have this new passport. It means a lot to me. Thank you again for your service." Roger felt a wave of relief pass through his body. Getting an American passport showing his current face was the first step in legitimizing his new life. "Now I can prove I'm American." They shook hands; Roger took a taxi back to the St. Regis and had a cup of coffee while he checked his email on his phone.

After a light lunch, he picked up his passport at the embassy, then went on to the lawyer's office in a very tall modern building. The lobby directory was in both English and Mandarin. When he checked in at the security desk, the attendant said, "Yes, Dr. Scully, they're expecting you. If you take the elevator to floor 38, they will greet you there." The entrance to the 38th floor resembled an upscale American law office. The receptionist stood up, greeted him by name, and immediately escorted him to a corner office, where she introduced him to Alfred Leung.

Leung said, "I understand you have a new passport. May I see it and your old passport?" He carefully inspected and returned them. Leung told Roger about Moon's investment in the transplant institute and the seven other Chinese research centers he supported. Roger shared with Leung his need to visit his parents, his budding surgical work at the lab, and his relationship with Lishan.

"Am I in danger of being deported? I need the medications I'm getting here," Roger asked.

"I understand, and we'll deal with your expired visa. How was your experience at the Institute?"

"They have treated me wonderfully well. I'm impressed by the skill and knowledge. I'm deeply indebted to them and your client for giving me a new life. It would never have occurred to me that someone could move my brain into a different body. Do you know what my body looked like before the transplant?"

"Not really. I understand that you lost your legs."

"More than my legs. The entire lower half of my body below the navel was gone. That operation is called a hemicorporectomy. Let me show you the picture." Roger pulled out his phone and displayed the picture of him naked, with pale lower body egg-shaped, devoid of penis and scrotum. A colostomy bag hung on the left abdomen and a urostomy bag on the right. Two lines of skin staples arced upward from the base around to his back on each side.

"I'm not sure I needed to see that, but I can see why you wanted something better."

"Of course. There are fewer than thirty cases reported in the literature. I couldn't face living like that, so I was glad to volunteer for Wong's program. I'm the only survivor of having my brain transplanted. Like Dr. Wong, I think of it as having a body transplanted to my brain."

"Amazing, amazing. Did you have any hesitation about accepting a body of another race?"

"I couldn't have. There was no Caucasian body available. After the transplant, the doctors put me into a coma for a few weeks. When I woke up, I had no idea what they had done. When I first saw myself in a mirror——well. I'm this blond Nordic-looking guy, and the person in the mirror is completely different. I screamed!"

Leung shook his head. "I cannot imagine your emotion or reaction. How about now?"

"I still do an occasional double-take when I pass a mirror. And now my girlfriend says I'm not truly Chinese. She calls me a Uyghur. I call myself an American."

"Well, you do have the Uyghur eyes, a longer nose, and lighter skin, but Americans don't have to worry about that. What are your career plans? When are you going back to the U.S.?"

"I need to go back to the States soon, even if for a short while, to tie up loose ends regarding my former life and to put my parents' minds at ease. I know I'll have to stay some months in Harbin for follow-up treatment. Also, I'm in a relationship with a young doctor in Harbin. She's about to start her surgical residency, and she may find it difficult to transfer her training to the U.S."

"I don't know anything about American immigration. I can refer you to a colleague if your friend needs help. Let's get you legal here for the moment. You're still a patient. So, you're not working at all?"

"I'm doing some surgery in the animal lab. They don't pay me, so it's part of my rehab."

"Make sure you don't get paid. Working for pay would be a quick way to get deported. Don't give immigration authorities any excuse to grab you."

"I may be interested in obtaining a job at the Institute, but I haven't talked to them about it. It would be nice to have a job, at least for the next year or so. My immediate problem is that expired visa; I'm living here illegally. I hope you'll be able to help me." Roger realized his hands were shaking. He had lived with an expired visa for two months. Since Ren had pointed out the situation, Roger had felt constantly stressed. If authorities discovered the situation, they would surely deport him.

"I'll have no problem getting you a new six-month visa," Leung assured him. "There's also a ten-year visa, which would allow you to work here. That's a little more complicated and can take a little longer to arrange. In either case, the usual bureaucratic process is daunting because you overstayed your previous visa. In these kinds of circumstances, we're better to avoid official channels and the paperwork required. A few calls to the right people and some lobbying on our part will expedite the process and make you legal."

At these words, Roger felt immediate relief. Others were representing him. They were avoiding official channels. *How does that work? Did someone pay a bribe?* He heard bribing officials was widespread in China. If Moon was making the payoff, it was not Zicheng's concern if it worked.

Leung continued, "Any visa you get will have certain limitations; foreigners are not free to go everywhere in this country. You're also subject to having your visa revoked if you violate its conditions or if U.S.-China relationships deteriorate. That latter prospect is quite possible and could result in your immediate deportation. A visitor in this country has no guarantees."

"Can I get a visa today? Now that I'm not in the hospital, I'm worried that I'll be picked up and deported as an illegal visitor."

Leung smiled, "Not to worry. No one will arrest you here. We should handle all the paperwork in a few days, and then you can return to Harbin as a legal person. You have a plane at your disposal for whatever day you want. Think it over tonight and come back tomorrow morning, when we'll work on whichever visa option you choose before meeting the Ministry officials in the afternoon. I understand the urgency of your position. You don't want to be living in this country illegally." With that, they decided to reconvene at 9 the following morning.

Roger lay on his back on his hotel bed, considering his options. The ten-year visa seemed best but might take longer to obtain. *How long will I stay in China? I haven't thought about that.* He had avoided the question of returning to Denver, where people would view him as a freaky celebrity. Boston would be the same. Whatever state he went to, he might face issues of medical qualification and board certification; he might even have to do a short residency to reconfirm his clinical skills after his surgery. The plus side would be accepting celebrity status and making money for a few years with speaking engagements and television appearances. He found that alternative unattractive. *Maybe I should stay and work in China for a year or so to sort things out. That means the ten-year visa. I'll have to get over the difficulties of working here speaking some Mandarin but being an American and not authentic Chinese.*

He should have thought through those professional problems before he had the surgery. He now remembered that the alternative of remaining a legless cripple had been utterly unacceptable. So, ultimately, he had concluded that he was better off to have the surgery and face unknown challenges rather than to live a life of despair in a partial body. He had made the right decision.

If the Colorado board knows about my surgery, they might not renew my medical license. I wonder if I could start a new life in Canada? They might accept my U.S. credentials without question or need for recertification. I should check that out. In the meantime, he had to decide which visa would be best. He leaned toward the ten-year because it would legalize his work at the Institute.

When he called Lishan that night, she was anxious to hear about his meetings in Beijing. He confirmed that he had obtained his new U.S. passport with no problems. "Lishan, the visa question will need another meeting tomorrow, but I think it's going to go well. This lawyer seems to know what he is doing and tells me I won't get arrested."

"Your new U.S. passport confirms your facial identity, but it's still as Roger Scully, not Wu Zicheng. What'll be the name on your new visa?"

"Since the visa will be in my passport, I assume it'll be for Roger Scully."

"Will the ten-year visa allow you to get a Chinese medical license?"

"I think so, but I don't know."

"How will you get a license? Could you practice away from Harbin?"

"Lishan, I told you I don't know all the details about the medical license."

And after some hesitation, she added, "With your new visa, can we marry?"

"Honey, I can't answer any of those questions right now. I'll keep them all in mind with my meetings today. Call you tomorrow night."

Roger was in Leung's office at 9 a.m. "I'll be happy to take a ten-year visa," he said solemnly.

"That is probably a wise decision," Leung acknowledged. "We have to do a little work on this; we will need your cooperation. As a first step, my assistant will help record your curriculum vitae and do some of the paperwork that will be required. When you have completed that, you will come back to me for more discussions." Leung pressed a button; almost immediately, a young man entered the room. "If you please, go with Kim, and he will get started on the paperwork."

In Kim's office, they sat at a table with some forms and a laptop computer. Kim said, "You'll see the laptop is set up for some routine questions. Please type your answers. I'm here to answer any questions." Roger went through the usual simple personal statistics and educational background. He listed his residency positions and his hospital appointment in Denver, as well as his specialist certification. Under hobbies, he reported hiking and skiing. "What is meant by the blank labeled political?" he asked.

"Are you a member of any political party?"

"No, I'm independent."

"In the United States, is independent a political party?" Kim asked.

"No, it means no political party."

"Then put no political party in the blank," said Kim. There were questions about previous arrests, drug use, psychiatric hospitalization, and organizational memberships. Roger had a clean record and listed his local medical association and the outdoor club in college. Under religion, he paused and then wrote Unitarian. He put his income level at the disability insurance level. Kim pressed a button and printed the completed questionnaire. He then took another sheet of paper from his folder and clipped it onto the form. It was a fingerprint sheet. "These are your fingerprints. We have them already."

Roger had a queasy feeling because he recalled no fingerprinting since leaving the U.S. However, authorities would have the body donor's prints from his prison experience. So, Roger's fingerprints had belonged to someone else. He shivered at the sudden realization. *Used fingerprints?* He was part Roger and part donor. His calloused hands had indicated heavy manual labor. His new body had some of the muscle memory of a person who had lived an entirely different life. That might explain how quickly he learned how to use chopsticks. He was aware that most muscle memory resided in the brain, but there was a muscle component. How would that affect Roger's future development?

The fingerprint issue triggered many of his recent concerns. The Scully gene pool had vanished; the family tree had come to an end. He was now living with genes from another family he knew nothing about. Roger felt momentarily dizzy at the question of being Chinese, American, or Uyghur. *I'm not sure I know who I am.*

Kim observed that Roger looked upset. "I think it is time for tea. You wait here, and I will get some." He reappeared a few minutes later with a small tray, a cup of tea, and pastries. Roger drank the tea but was not hungry. They returned to Leung, who explained that his office would forward all the information to a senior official, who likely would want to meet Roger soon. "I'll make some calls and see if it is possible for the meeting to be this week. If not, then you're free to return to Harbin this afternoon. Wait in your hotel for my call." They shook hands, and Roger returned to the St. Regis. A few hours later, Leung called and said, "This week is not possible. We are trying for a meeting late next week, so you'll have to return to Harbin. You will have your customary transportation. Will that be all right?"

"Of course. Is there anything I need to prepare?"

"No preparation is necessary. However, I suggest you polish your Mandarin. I will see you when you return here."

"Thank you very much, Leung." He noticed he already had an email message that his flight would depart at 4 pm. He called Lishan and arranged to meet her at Wuxiaomei Barbecue, their favorite restaurant. The return flight was uneventful. The officials at the airport accepted his new U.S. passport without comment. During the flight, for several minutes, he stared at his new U.S. passport photo. *Yes, I'm officially American.*

At their reunion, Lishan was excited but also looked worried. In a quiet corner of the restaurant, he showed her the new U.S. passport. Lishan said, "So in your pocket, you are Roger, and sitting here, you are Zicheng."

"That's correct," he answered. He then explained the prospect of the long-term visa and how he'd come to his decision. He also mentioned he would have to return to Beijing next week for an interview.

"The long-term visa will be wonderful. We can live and work anywhere in the country. But how do I fit into this equation? I'm still feeling a little insecure. I worry that if you get back to the States, I'll never see you again. You never discuss my career, as though it doesn't matter. We have to look at what I do when I finish my residency."

"I'm sorry. I was preoccupied with my situation. We need to work on your career plans. You're the reason I'm applying for a long-term visa. I need to visit my parents soon, but that'll be just a short trip. I can't bear the thought of leaving you here with me moving back to live in the States. I live here now. The long-term visa and working here is the best answer."

With tears streaming down her face, she said, "Roger, I mean Zicheng, I love you—thank you, thank you, thank you."

CHAPTER 10

The morning after his return from Beijing, Zicheng reported to the laboratory in his scrubs. Li said, "We've lots of work for you to do. Wait until you see the schedule." Zicheng explained that he would probably have to leave for one day for a second interview in Beijing. Li understood and said they would work around his schedule. In the meantime, he wanted Zicheng to do more advanced work on the gorillas. Two days later, Zicheng removed the right foot of one gorilla. He then assisted in reattaching it to the ankle of another gorilla. The surgery with Wong, Li, and Zicheng all participating took eight hours. Zicheng was exhausted but happy that he had performed well in surgery nearly as intricate as a brain transplant. He was a surgeon again.

After, Li said, "This was a test for you. We needed to see how you worked, especially on some of the finer connections. Now I have a surprise. Next week we're doing a human transplant, and it's on your friend Ke. You'll be on the team for that surgery. Because you'll be the second assistant on my team, you won't have much responsibility. Wong's team will be opening Ke, while you and I will open the donor.

After we remove the donor's brain, you can stand aside and watch while I join Wong's team for the actual transplant of Ke's brain into the donor. When that transplant is over, you'll join the surgical team removing Ke's organs from the old body for use in other transplants. You'll have a very long day."

"Oh, my God," Zicheng exclaimed. "You're giving me a great opportunity. I will do my best."

"Ke does not know the date of the surgery yet. We'll tell him shortly. In the meantime, say nothing to anyone about our plans. Just as when you had your surgery, you didn't know most of the surgical team. And we'll keep it that way."

Over the next two days, Wong, Li, and Zicheng rehearsed the surgery, using 3-D printed brain replicas of Ke and skull basins identical to the donor. Zicheng was amazed at the feeling of reality, operating on the artificial tissues that closely resembled the brain's appearance and texture. As they worked, Zicheng commented, "My God, these brains do everything but bleed."

"And think," replied Wong.

Am I going to be operating on someone who has become such a friend? After much thought, he decided it was an honor to help him.

That night Zicheng said to Lishan, "Next week Ke gets his transplant. And guess what? I'm on the team."

"Wow, that's exciting. What does Ke think?"

"He doesn't even know about the date yet, and we won't tell him I am on the team."

"I understand. I'm proud that you're part of the surgical team. You have come so far."

"I have my confidence back. That's important. Let's talk about something else. I'm tired of living in the cottage. It's time for us to find an apartment. I don't need to live in a hospital setting anymore, and if we find a place near the hospital, it'll be handy for both of us. What do you think?"

Lishan, surprised at the suggestion, grinned widely. Zicheng could see that she liked the idea of leaving the cramped cottage. She said, "That sounds wonderful. I had been thinking about it, but I hesitated to ask you. So, your idea is great for me. I'll start the search tomorrow. I think I know who to ask."

"I know nothing about finding or renting an apartment in this country, so it's going to be in your hands. Don't sign anything, though, until I have the next interview in Beijing. That should clarify my status, but we can start looking now."

That evening, Zicheng and Lishan attended a Chinese opera at the stunning Harbin Opera House, a structure that attracted international attention because of its architecture. Zicheng marveled at the sinuous building reflecting the wilderness and cold climate surrounding the city. He had read of the 850,000 square foot interior, the two theaters, and many innovative architectural features. Looking up, he compared the heavy timber beams to those he had seen in the grand Adirondack lodges.

Unlike any of the few opera performances Zicheng had attended in Boston and New York, the opera was a noisy spectacular. Performers had elaborate costumes, including fanciful headdresses. In lieu of an orchestra, a collection of drummers and a few string instruments plied the pentatonic scale. As a musician, Zicheng found that scale vaguely troubling, like everything done in a minor key. Unlike American audiences, the Harbin spectators were animated, raucous when they sang along with some arias.

After the performance, Lishan asked, "Well, what do you think of Chinese opera?"

"I never developed any taste for Western opera. I'm not sure I will be a fan of the Chinese version. But it's fun for a night."

"I don't think you like Chinese culture very much."

"I disagree. I love Kung Fu, Chinese acrobats, and architecture like this. Give me more time. Remember, I wasn't born into this culture."

Wong had scheduled Ke's surgery for three days later. That night, an email came in from Leung with Zicheng's Beijing interview appointment three days after Ke's operation. There would be the usual arrangements for the plane and hotel. Zicheng and Lishan went to bed and talked excitedly about Zicheng's progress with his documents and developing surgical skills.

Ke shared his news that he was about to have his surgery within the week. Zicheng tried to reassure him and explained the puzzlement he would feel on awakening. Zicheng called out, "Fong, bring us a round of beers to celebrate Ke's news."

Although Ke was excited and reassured by Zicheng's previous success, he was also apprehensive. "It went well for you, Zicheng, but I'm scared shitless," Ke said. "When I signed up for the program, I never believed the operation would happen."

Sung spoke up. "If the operation doesn't work, you never wake up. If it works, you wake up like Zicheng did."

"I guess you're right, but I think I need another beer," Ke said.

"By the time you're finished, the surgeons will have worked out all the bugs for my operation. I'm glad they have you to practice on," said Sung with a smile.

As had happened with Zicheng, Ke moved from the cottage to the hospital the day before his surgery. Zicheng did not reveal his participation with the surgical team. Zicheng was in a conference room for the pre-op meeting; he did not see Ke depart.

Zicheng sat in the crowded room, listening intently. Dr. Wong stood in front of a team of about twenty specialized surgery staff, speaking in Mandarin. "Thank you for coming. We are on the eve of another significant event in transplant science. We will now prepare our checklists for eighteen hours of surgery. Remember, in making the lists, think of everything that might go wrong. We must respond quickly. We need to prepare for both the surgery and post-op care. Since we expect up to two weeks of hypothermia and coma, you three anesthesiologists will be responsible for continuous monitoring and controlling respiration and temperature during and after the operation.

"Operating room nurses and technicians, you will work with Dr. Li to walk through the operations we are planning. You must anticipate every step; list all of your equipment requirements. PLAN FOR REDUNDANCY. If an instrument falls to the floor, you will have another ready.

"Careful post-op care is vital to our success. You must visit the patient several times a day. You will use your massage techniques to keep limbs moving and skin healthy. We cannot have bed sores or stiff joints. Dr. Bin now has a few words."

Dr. Bin faced the audience. "You may wonder what a psychiatrist has to do with surgery. Let me explain. I'm concerned about brain function, especially after something as traumatic as being moved into another skull. We anticipate a period when most brain functions shut down. After the shock, there must be recovery. Don't think that just because our patient Ke is in a coma from drugs, his brain is not working." As Zicheng listened, he recalled his coma, with its Chinese voices and weird sounds. And the reading of *Love Story*. "So, around the patient, watch what you say. He may hear you, even while unconscious. Don't make loud noises that might frighten him. Be gentle when you move him, and explain beforehand what you are about to do.

"Most of you have heard of diurnal rhythms, the body's response to the time of day. The surgery might abolish those rhythms, so we need to re-establish them. I want the hours of 2200 to 0600 to be quiet and dark. During the day, I want daylight streaming into the room. Controlling light and noise should help Ke restore his diurnal rhythms. Finally, let me congratulate all of you for being chosen to participate in this important treatment advance. His post-op care may make the difference between success and failure.

"Understand that post-op, he will be very confused. At first, he will not know what surgery he has had. He will be shocked to see that his face is one he has never seen before. All of the previous patients said their first look in a mirror was the most difficult moment in the recovery."

Zicheng, standing at the back of the room, nodded as he remembered the moment. *Bin said previous patients. I guess that means me and the two earlier "volunteers."*

Wong resumed his position. "Split yourselves into teams to plan the surgery and recovery. Feel free to communicate and cooperate with other teams. Post-op nurses and massage therapists need to talk to the anesthesiologists about rotating or moving the patient. Remember, this is a team effort. Thank you."

Zicheng had been listening with fascination. He had not appreciated the preparation and number of people involved in his previous surgery. They scheduled to go from the opening to closing in eighteen hours, but Wong and Zicheng realized that unforeseen delays could make it longer. Therefore, they included toilet and refreshment breaks in the plans for each team member.

At 6 a.m. the day of Ke's surgery, Zicheng was aware of nurses wheeling two sedated patients into the oversize operating room during his twenty-minute scrub. He was aware of his stress level. *I think my pulse rate is over 100, and it's a good thing no one is taking my blood pressure.*

When the surgeons entered the room, they saw two operating tables. Each had an unconscious patient sitting upright, bald head shining under the lights as a nurse scrubbed, then applied disinfection. Once the surgery started, every member of the team focused on following the precise operative plan. The two teams worked simultaneously, doing similar things on both Ke and the donor.

Bovie knives burned through the scalps with the typical smell of burning grease when they reached the subcutaneous fat layer. On each exposed skull, the saws' small oscillating blade smoothly sliced through to the brain cavity.

CLANG! Several of the team jerked upright; Wong had just tossed Ke's discarded skull top into a metal basin. Another hour passed in almost complete silence.

"Ready over here, Dr. Wong," said Li.

"Okay, clear that skull and then come over here."

Li tightened all his ligatures and made a quick scalpel slice under the donor's brain. A nurse presented him with a basin into which he tossed the mushy mass he had lifted from the donor's head. He moved to the area behind Ke's skull and, at a nod from Wong, sliced the spinal cord-to-brain junction.

Everyone present held their breath as Wong lifted Ke's brain out of the skull and carried it in both hands for a few steps to the other gurney. With Li cradling the head, Wong slipped the pale brain into the donor's cranial cavity. Tension left the room like water down a drain. Hours of delicate work followed to connect the arteries and veins, using the robotic microscope. To nerves and spinal cord, the surgeons applied a paste of polyethylene glycol, a common laxative. Li used the English term "glue" when he requested it from the scrub nurse. These procedures, mostly robotic, were demanding but more routine. At the end of the surgery, the new Ke was unconscious, on a ventilator, and had stable vital signs. He went to the recovery room in good condition.

Zicheng was awestruck and tired from the effort of the day-long procedure and the tension. Now he accompanied the brainless body to an adjoining OR where another surgical team stood waiting. With swift and deliberate movements, surgeons cut the corneas, kidneys, lungs, heart, and liver from the corpse. The corneas would restore sight to a blind teenager. The kidneys relieved two men from the travail of chronic renal dialysis. The lungs replaced the failing lungs of a twenty-four-year-old with cystic fibrosis. Another team transplanted the heart into a thirty-one-year-old mother with chronic myocarditis and heart failure. They gave her children their mom back. Finally, Ke's liver saved two children with chronic liver failure. Seven more persons had benefited from Ke's transplant. After all the organ extractions and draining of the remaining blood supply into storage bags, an attendant wheeled the emptied body to the morgue.

Exhausted, Zicheng reflected on the day's events. He had witnessed and participated in the procedure that had given him new life only weeks before. *I never imagined I would be part of this procedure. Wow!*

Two days later, Zicheng visited Ke, who now lay unconscious in the familiar room with the Mandarin plaque. After a brief chat with the anesthesiologist, Zicheng left feeling optimistic for Ke. That evening, he shared the good news with Lishan, Sung, and Fong.

CHAPTER 11

Zicheng's second trip to Beijing was uneventful. He arrived at dinner time, checked into the St. Regis, and had a perfectly made cocktail and dinner. The following morning, Leung picked him up at the hotel entrance. During their half-hour drive, he briefed him on what to expect. Leung said, "You will meet three people. I suggest you greet them in Mandarin, although they will probably ask questions in English to facilitate the interview. They have scheduled two hours for the meeting. I am not sure of everything that will happen because I cannot ask too many questions of senior officials. They might bring up the question of Chinese citizenship. They may ask if you want to consider that, but you'd have to renounce your U.S. citizenship."

Roger blanched at the thought. *Give up my American citizenship?* He had assumed that born American, he would die American, no matter what happened to his body. *Why did Leung mention Chinese citizenship?* He had never considered, let alone asked for, citizenship.

They soon arrived at an imposing government-looking building with armed guards at each side of the entrance. A video camera at the doorway focused on each face. In China, facial recognition is ubiquitous. Once inside, Leung presented his ID card and the Roger Scully passport, which a security guard scanned. A young man in a dark suit appeared within a few seconds, nodded, and said, "Please follow me," in Mandarin. He took them to a small conference room, where three Chinese gentlemen, all about sixty years old, were seated at a round table. Each had a black leather folder. Leung managed the introductions in Mandarin.

The man in the center of the three, Lao Xing, smiled before addressing them in English. "Thank you for coming, Dr. Wu Zicheng. You are a unique person with whom we look forward to having a continuing relationship. Your story represents a major medical advance of which China can be rightfully proud. I understand that you have made an excellent recovery and currently work as a surgeon at the Institute. Am I correct?"

"Yes, sir," Zicheng said. "Dr. Wong has kindly allowed me to train with his surgical team. I'm honored to work with him and his colleagues."

For the next hour, the five discussed Wu Zicheng's plans if he stayed in China. When he mentioned Lishan, it was clear from the nods that they already knew about her. He did not discuss the idea of Lishan doing a surgical residency in the United States. Zicheng explained, "Originally, I intended to return to the United States as soon as I recovered. I have now rethought that plan; I see more issues concerning medical licensure and publicity in America. I am interested in working with the team in Harbin. Frankly, I am somewhat muddled about my future."

The three Chinese officials looked at each other in agreement.

"You might not have thought of becoming a Chinese citizen," said Lao Xing, "but we would like you to consider that, so you could live and work here. Usually, a foreigner must renounce his country's citizenship to become a Chinese citizen. We have pondered over this issue in preparing for this meeting. We have come up with a proposal for your consideration." They all noted Roger's involuntary stiffening and his frown at this opening.

After a long pause, he continued, "Consider this scenario: you are now Wu Zicheng, born in Harbin on January 8, 1985. You are not converting from foreign citizenship. With the necessary documents authenticating this new birth date, you will be like any other China-born citizen with the same rights and responsibilities. There is no need to reference either your surgery or your previous history. What do you think of that?"

Zicheng was startled at this unexpected proposal. "Are you really offering me Chinese citizenship? And more than that, you are suggesting a new identity. What do I do about my U.S. citizenship and passport?"

"Well, that is up to Roger Scully, who is not here today. We are talking to Wu Zicheng and not Roger Scully. Roger Scully may continue to exist in the eyes of the U.S. government bureaucracy, but that is not our affair. If there is a Roger Scully in American records, it is of no interest to us," said Lao Xing.

"Could I please speak alone for a few minutes with my attorney?" Zicheng asked. With that, they retreated into a smaller room where an attendant offered tea, which they accepted.

"God Almighty, it sounds like a perfect solution if I can get away with it. What problems do you see, Leung?"

"We must ascertain what conditions, if any, will apply. I would be particularly concerned about foreign travel and your right to work, which would include medical licensure. We should also check that there are no marriage restrictions, although I can't imagine any."

"I need to understand this. Are these officials saying I can have two identities?"

"I don't see any other interpretation. They consider Wu Zicheng a person separate from Roger Scully. You seem to lose nothing."

"Then I'll go for it. I'll gladly accept the citizenship offer."

Leung nodded, then rang a small bell. An attendant escorted them back to the conference room.

Leung opened the discussion. "My client needs to know if he will have any foreign travel restrictions."

Lao Xing answered, "Like any Chinese citizen, he is free to travel abroad. We have only one condition. We would ask that you notify us of all foreign travel and the duration of any foreign stay. It is not an issue of getting permission, but we need to be informed. We would also ask to be notified of any travel and stay planned by Dr. Roger Scully."

Roger's brain dinged at hearing the mention of dual identities. He still became momentarily confused when confronted with his duality. *Am I Roger, or am I Zicheng?*

Leung continued, "Dr. Wu is concerned about his right to work and practice medicine in this country."

One of the other gentlemen spoke up and pointed out that he controlled all medical licensure. If Wu Zicheng wished to work as a doctor in China, he would arrange for the necessary credentials and explain what authorities would expect of him. In the meantime, Wu Zicheng could continue to work as an assistant surgeon at the Harbin Institute.

In response to Leung's question about marriage, it was clear there was no restriction. When asked about any other conditions of the arrangement, Lao Xing replied, "As I said earlier, Wu Zicheng represents a major achievement in Chinese medicine. Once Dr. Wong publishes the paper on his scientific work, the world will appreciate more the medical advances in the Republic of China. We expect Dr.

Wu will make himself available to the media in China and possibly elsewhere. His story will not divulge anything of his history before the operation, except his training as a doctor. After a few months of publicity, I would expect that the press and others will find other stories to chase. Is that condition agreeable?"

Zicheng answered, "I have previously not liked the idea of being a media target. Further, it sounds as if I will exist with two identities, which is confusing. But considering all the challenges I will face, this would be the least I could do to repay Dr. Wong and everyone else for what they did for me. I gratefully accept your offer to become a Chinese citizen. Thank you, thank you."

Lao Xing arose, "Gentlemen, I think that concludes our meeting for today. Mr. Leung, if you and Dr. Wu could return here tomorrow morning with passport photos, we will be able to take care of all of the paperwork. By tomorrow evening, the doctor will have his new passport, and he can return to doing surgery."

On the return ride to the hotel, Zicheng was practically speechless. The solution seemed so simple and workable. *I never would've thought this. What kind of government could create a new person? Maybe this was the Chinese equivalent of the witness protection program.* When dropped at the hotel, he started to offer profuse thanks to Leung, who interrupted, "Dr. Wu, don't thank me. Thank Dr. Wong at the Institute and the People's Republic of China. I will call and let you know what time I'll pick you up tomorrow."

Back in his room, Zicheng immediately called Lishan, "You won't believe this, but tomorrow I'll be a Chinese citizen. Find that apartment."

"Citizen?' Lishan asked, incredulous. "You're not kidding me?"

"No, I'm serious. And I'm going to get my medical license as well."

"This is wonderful and incredible news. I never imagined

citizenship. I'll look for the apartment tomorrow. Can we celebrate when you get back?"

"Of course. We have a lot to celebrate." After the call, Zicheng pondered the events of the day. Senior Chinese officials could create citizens without qualms over laws or policies. He assumed that Mr. Moon or his agent had paid a bribe. He would become a Chinese citizen without forfeiting U.S. citizenship. Zicheng was astounded but foresaw significant complications if the U.S. government learned of this arrangement. It appeared he legally would be both Roger Scully and Wu Zicheng, with two identities and separate citizenships in two countries. He could hardly believe this was happening. *I feel like an actor in a spy film. Is it all too simple?*

The following morning, Leung drove him to the photography shop for the pictures, then back to the government office. The same minor official from the previous day greeted them, examined the photos, and assured them the passport would be ready in two hours. As they left, Leung said, "I'll take you back to the hotel so you can check out and have lunch. Then we'll pick up your passport and go to the airport. My office has booked you on a regular commercial flight this afternoon to Harbin. Your new passport will serve as your identification."

Zicheng went through the next few hours feeling like he was in a dream. In the departure lounge, he stared at his new passport. Then, after ensuring that no one could see him, he compared the Chinese document to his recent United States version.

Lishan greeted him at the airport, in her best dress, with an armful of flowers. "Congratulations, my wonderful Wu Zicheng, the new Chinese citizen. I'm so excited."

"I had trouble believing it would happen, but it did. Thank God I'm now legal."

"I found an apartment for us. It's within walking distance of the hospital and is almost a new building. Tomorrow morning we have an appointment with the landlord. You might think it's too expensive, but I picked the two-bedroom one to have a room for an office we can share."

"You helped me get to this place with all your work and support this past year. Now we can relax and enjoy life. It's a huge relief to be legal and able to get on with my life." They went to dinner, drank too much wine, and kept Sung awake with their bedtime activity.

In the morning, Lishan led him to an unpretentious, sparsely furnished second-floor apartment. Zicheng found the rooms small, by American standards. As he checked out the tiny balcony off the bedroom, he heard Lishan and the landlord in a kitchen conversation. The landlord's voice was indistinct, but Lishan's voice was loud and direct, "What do you mean Uyghur! He is a Han doctor."

The landlord suddenly sounded apologetic at his mistake. Zicheng was uncertain whether the term *Han* was more important than the word *doctor*, but it was clear they could rent the apartment. Within minutes, Wu Zicheng signed the lease for one year. They completed the deal with a check written by Lishan.

As they were leaving, Zicheng said, "Lishan, now I can open a bank account and repay your rent deposit. I can even get a Chinese credit card. What was the disagreement about me being a Uyghur?"

"Don't worry about it. When that man saw you, he told me that he does not rent to Uyghurs. That's my bank across the street. Because they know me, there should be no problems."

"Should I expect to be always discriminated against because I look Uyghur?"

"I took care of it. Don't overreact."

Zicheng ended the discussion, unsatisfied.

Within minutes after entering the bank, Zicheng had a passbook and a checkbook. He had instructions on how to wire funds from the U.S. and assurances that the bank would issue his credit card upon receipt of the U.S. funds.

With his last barrier to Chinese legal status cleared, Zicheng felt much relief. Lishan was studying hard for her final exams before graduation in two months. He was now spending two or three days each week in the hospital OR and working the other days in the Institute. Soon he was speaking what he called "operating room Mandarin" because of his continued contact with OR teams. His sixty-hour workweek was typical for Chinese surgeons.

Within the month, he tendered his American credentials. A week later, the Chinese government sent him his medical license (suitable for framing) with a wallet-size duplicate. With some delight, he showed his license card to Dr. Wong. "Now, I am what we call in the U.S. street legal."

"Congratulations, Zicheng. We have been anticipating this day. I have a surprise for you," he said as he reached for a parcel near his desk. He surprised Zicheng by handing over the paper-wrapped bundle. "You may open it."

Zicheng ripped open the flimsy paper wrapping to find a neatly folded long white laboratory coat of the type worn by the professors, medical staff, and teaching fellows. He broke into a broad grin on seeing embroidered above the left breast pocket, *Wu Zicheng, MD,* in both Chinese and English characters. He had rejoined his profession.

The following day, he wore his new coat to surgical transplant rounds. Dr. Wong and another professor led a gaggle of staff, residents, and medical students down the corridor, discussing cases and occasionally examining a patient. Zicheng was pleased that Lishan, a student in the group, exhibited no recognition of him during rounds. The teaching routine in a Harbin hospital was the same as at an American hospital. Before returning to the laboratory, Zicheng took the elevator to visit Ke in the secure unit. At Ke's door, a set of signs indicated, in Mandarin, "No admittance. Infection Protocol Required. Authorized personnel only."

When he opened the door, a nurse, masked and swathed in protective gear, stopped him at the entrance. "I am sorry, doctor, but you cannot enter." He retreated and returned to the laboratory, where he immediately sought out Li.

"Li, what's happening with Ke?"

"Massive fungal infection, we think. We're trying some new drugs, but it doesn't look good. Don't tell Sung about this."

"Okay, but please keep me informed. I feel lucky that I escaped that complication. Since they won't let me into his room, you're my only source of information." A sense of sadness overtook Zicheng as he realized the likely inevitability of his friend's death. Both men were silent for several minutes while they examined the gorillas' wounds. The tension was palpable.

"What did you think of rounds today?" Li asked.

"I noticed that kidneys are the most common organs transplanted here, which did not surprise me. But why are so many of the patients Arab?"

Li replied, "You're correct that kidney transplants are the most common of our transplant procedures. Fortunately, we have the world's largest supply of donors. Arabs come here because they have the money, and their home countries have relatively few donors. Harbin even has a small hotel near the hospital for Arabs awaiting transplants. There is a dialysis center right in the hotel to maintain them while they wait."

"Don't Chinese waiting for kidneys get upset at Arabs getting available organs?"

"No, you do not understand. We assign donor organs to recipients based on patients' needs. We do not deprive Chinese citizens of transplants. Arabs sometimes have to wait many weeks in their hotel. That said, many Chinese kidneys now live in the Middle East."

"Do you also have donors who are not prisoners?"

"We have a few of those, usually the siblings of the patients. We are fortunate to have an ample supply of prisoner donors, unlike you in America."

Zicheng nodded his understanding as he marveled at a system that produced a supply of kidneys sufficient to create a surplus for export. He gulped at the thought of so many executed persons. He asked, "Do you think it's right to kill so many people?"

"That is not my concern. I am not a lawyer. These prisoners have been tried and found guilty. They agree to donate organs; My role is to benefit the persons needing organs." Li's shrug indicated the end of the discussion, leaving Zicheng with his thoughts.

Zicheng was surprised to receive a text with an appointment for an audiogram. He approached Li. "Why am I booked for a hearing test? My tinnitus disappeared."

Li explained, "Dr. Wong is still evaluating your recovery, and we need to know about all your cranial nerves. Your pre-op audiogram showed some noise-induced hearing loss, probably from playing rock music. It'll be interesting to see what your pattern looks like now. You'll also be getting another eye exam."

"But the ophthalmology department saw me in hospital and gave me the prescription for glasses."

"But we want to go further than that. They will check your visual fields. Don't you remember having them done during your work-up?"

"Oh, yeah, sitting in that machine waiting for lights to appear. I remember that one."

"We're trying to document, as much as possible, all your neurologic functions. We'll probably end up publishing a series of papers on you." Zicheng felt like a biology specimen in a laboratory that considered prisoners as a commodity and patients as part of a grand experiment.

CHAPTER 12

Zicheng continued to improve his physical condition. Every morning before work, he participated in a Tai Chi class at the hospital. Lishan declined to join him. At the end of the workday, he used the hospital gym for an hour of aerobics and weight training. He visited Harbin's indoor ski facility (the world's largest); it was crowded and devoid of any appeal. Next year, he would try skiing at one of the many outdoor ski resorts near Harbin.

On one of his Institute days, Li took him aside and handed him a manuscript typed in English. Li explained, "This is the paper we are submitting to the journal *Lancet* concerning you and your operation. We have been careful to do nothing that might identify you. But if the paper is published, there will soon be publicity in China and elsewhere. We must be careful not to share this paper until it is published." Zicheng read the paper carefully. The short case report described his transplant after what the authors described as a massive injury. They made no mention of the previous hemicorporectomy. The article identified the patient as a doctor who had now been able to return to full function. There was no mention of the donor source.

The paper was authored by doctors Wong and Li.

That evening, when he shared the paper with Lishan, she was excited, "Zicheng, you're going to be famous!"

"I hope not. Wong and Li warned that this would happen. And at some point, they'll present me as the specimen. It was part of my agreement with the Chinese government, but they have assured me of confidentiality concerning my original identity. We'll stick to my made-up story about being raised in the U.S. by Chinese parents. We hope that the U.S. press doesn't try to find an American medical graduate called Wu Zicheng. I'd feel more comfortable if I made my visit back to Boston before the paper is published. Tomorrow I'll meet with Wong and ask for a ten-day leave to make that trip. In the meantime, remember I was not to show this to anyone, so keep the paper confidential."

Lishan nodded, "You're the best one to decide on the trip. I'll be busy with my exams for the next few weeks, anyway, but I'll still miss you." Zicheng suspected that she was concerned lest he would decide not to come back.

The next day he obtained permission for the time off. Wong was pleased that Zicheng was taking great pains to preserve confidentiality. That same day, Zicheng made his airline reservation to fly to Hong Kong as Wu Zicheng. After confirming that leg of his journey, he immediately reserved round-trip business class flights for Roger Scully from Hong Kong to Boston. His use of two different names, his Chinese and his American visa credit cards, and his two different email accounts, meant no one could link one flight to the other. That evening, he called his parents to inform them of his travel plans. He stressed the need for confidentiality due to the impending publication. He swore them to secrecy concerning his visit. He then emailed them his itinerary. He also copied Leung so that he might notify the Chinese officials.

Discussing the U.S. visit with Lishan, Zicheng said, "I wish you were coming with me. I'd love for you to get to know my parents and to see Boston and perhaps other parts of America. After we get over the publicity interval, we should be able to travel much more easily. In the meantime, let's try to keep your identity and our relationship out of any press coverage."

"Yes, keep me out of it for now. I don't want my family to see my name in the paper or on television. I still have to figure out a way to deal with my parents and our relationship."

Zicheng was not looking forward to the many hours of flying. From Harbin to Hong Kong was eight hours. Hong Kong to Boston was about another twenty hours. He arranged to stay overnight in a Hong Kong airport hotel before starting the longer leg of the journey.

On the day before his departure, Wong invited him to his office, where he announced, "*Lancet* will publish the paper in a month to six weeks. I've had considerable correspondence with their editor. Their first reaction was to reject the paper on ethical grounds. After I argued with them, they decided to publish along with two commentaries they invited from well-known medical ethicists. One will be harsh and denounce our operation as unethical experimentation. I think the other will be more supportive. In any case, they're publishing us, and I'm sure there will be many letters to the editor after the publication. I'm happy that you'll be back here when this happens, so you'll have input into our responses. In the meantime, enjoy your trip. We look forward to your return—you're an important part of the team."

When Zicheng packed, he included a copy of the manuscript. He considered his timing of the U.S. trip to be fortuitous, given the *Lancet* response. The night before his departure, Zicheng and Lishan had dinner at their favorite restaurant and made love tenderly before he caught his morning taxi to the airport. There was no problem with his identification in boarding the Harbin to Hong Kong flight as Wu Zicheng. He used his Roger Scully identification and credit cards at the airport hotel. With his American passport, he quickly cleared departure security and U.S. customs and immigration. In the hotel and on the long overseas flight, he found it strange and pleasant to hear so much English spoken.

At Logan Airport, Roger immediately spotted his parents but saw they looked anxious. Although they had visited him in Harbin, they looked a little questioningly at this Chinese man approaching them. When he opened his arms, his parents embraced Roger with no reservation.

"Is this really you?" his mother asked. She was smiling and crying at the same time. "I thought I'd never get you back here. I was so worried. And now here you are looking strong and well. You've gained some weight since we saw you in the hospital. It's wonderful to have you home again." His father withdrew from the hug and smiled.

As Roger described his flight to Boston, his mother interrupted him. "Oh, Roger, you look different, but the way you speak is the same, your smile is the same, and your shrug is the same, so you're my old Roger." Roger grinned and gave her an extra hug.

Since they had previously endured the same long flights from Boston to Harbin and back, they fully understood Roger's fatigue. He was also struggling with the twelve-hour time change. They wanted to show him to their closest friends and senior people at the restaurant; Roger emphasized that they needed to protect his identity. With publicity about to break, there was every reason to keep his secret. "There'll be a time in the future when we may be more public," said Roger. "In the meantime, please, please, keep our secret and work with me on this. Let's just enjoy our visit."

Once home in Natick, he gratefully collapsed in his old room and instantly fell asleep. When he awakened a few hours later, he went to the kitchen, headed straight for the cupboard beside the refrigerator, and withdrew a canister. "I see you still remember where the cookies are," Mildred smiled. Roger was pleased to see that his mother had prepared all his favorite dishes, and he felt comfortable sitting with them at the familiar dining table.

His parents wanted to hear every detail about his life in China. He had to describe his work, his apartment, and, of course, his plans regarding Lishan. They insisted he should take back to her a graduation gift from them.

He had informed them of his Chinese legal status. "This will come as a surprise to you. I am now a Chinese citizen."

"A what? You gave up your American citizenship?" asked his father.

He proceeded with a detailed explanation of his process with the Chinese officials and the resulting dual citizenship. Mildred looked puzzled and asked, "Will that ever stop you from coming home?"

"No, Mom. The U.S. government isn't aware of my Chinese citizenship, and I doubt the Chinese are likely to tell them. I think I have the best of situations. I can continue to work in Harbin during my treatment. I can come back to the States whenever I want. I'm still an American citizen."

His father looked skeptical. "You shouldn't trust them so much."

"I'm just being realistic. It seems they've bent over backward to help you out since the surgery. The passport, the citizenship, and the medical license. They'll want something from you down the line."

"Dad, they've kept their word on everything so far. Please don't be racist."

"I'm just being realistic. You can't trust Asians from anywhere."

Roger sighed and declined to continue the argument.

Although they understood Roger's need to remain in China for treatment, they expressed concern about his eventual return to the

U.S. Surely, they said, he wasn't considering living in China permanently. He did not answer that question.

His week in Boston passed quickly. He was delighted to see two Red Sox games at Fenway Park and dined with his parents at Locke Ober's. He did not contact any of his friends or classmates. In the mail that his parents had not yet forwarded was a notice from the Colorado Medical Board. His license was due for renewal.

Along with that notice was a form for him to list his continuing medical education particulars and credits. Over the past year, he had fulfilled his continuing education courses by completing the *New England Journal of Medicine* online exercises. Since the Board seemed unaware of his disability claim, he would renew his license with a Natick address.

When it was time to leave, with Mildred in tears, Roger suggested they have a reunion soon, not in Harbin, but somewhere more glamorous, like Hong Kong or Singapore. All three cried as they said goodbye at Logan Airport.

On the return flight, he had felt queasy about the forthcoming publicity. He again stayed at the Hong Kong airport hotel; the next day changed passports for the flight to Harbin. All uneventful. He had transitioned from Zicheng to Roger and back with no problem with travel or immigration officials. He had much preferred being Roger instead of Zicheng. He had enjoyed hearing English all the time. He felt more Roger than Zicheng.

Lishan welcomed him warmly. "I'm so glad you're back. How was the visit with your parents?"

"It was great. They were more comfortable with me at home than they were at the hospital. They've accepted their new son. What are you doing about your trip home?"

"The day after graduation, I'll go home for a week. I'm not comfortable living in the village, since I've spent most of my life in the city. Then I'll have a few weeks to rest up before I start on the residency. We can still do our tour of the country."

"Do they know about me yet?"

"No, I have to discuss that when I see them. It's going to be a hard sell. I was always the gold medal student, the honor to the family and the village, and all that. They're very conservative. It'll be one issue that we are living together, another if they find out you're an American."

"Would it help if I went with you?"

"God, no. I have to do it alone. Let's talk about something happy. Can we still take that vacation we were planning?"

"I'll work with Li to get the time off."

"You won't see very much of me when I start working."

"Been there, done that—if it's anything like American residency, I'll understand." He nodded. "But first, let's deal with graduation. Let me buy you an extra special dress for the big event. For a change, you are going to get something glamorous and expensive," he insisted. "And, further, here's a present from my parents." He presented her with a neatly wrapped small gift with a perfectly tied ribbon.

Lishan gasped when she opened the packet. There, in a small satin-lined box, was a fiery opal pendant on a gold chain. "Oh my God, it's beautiful." Roger recognized the locket as a prized piece from his mother's collection of antique jewelry. He nodded approval, pleased with his mother's choice.

"I'm going to email her a thank-you right now," which she did.

The *Lancet* published Wong's article the day before Lishan's graduation in Chengdu on May 24. Zicheng continued to work at the Institute, which was under siege from the media. CNN not only covered the story but also sent a reporter to Harbin. Zicheng watched the clip about it that his parents emailed to him. A reporter wearing gold-rimmed glasses looked wide-eyed at the camera as she read the report. "A team of Chinese surgeons is reporting a successful *brain* transplant. You heard me correctly. This never-before procedure appeared in the *Lancet*—"

The body transplant was a worldwide sensation. Almost every major newspaper ran the story in both the States and China. Zicheng collected the articles but had trouble reading them; they filled him with concern. His fears intensified when the reporters began showing up. Three days after the *Lancet* published, he first noticed them. They stood outside of the hospital in the morning with the particular stance—weary and wary at the same time—of journalists. The press naturally wanted to interview Wong, but more importantly, hoped to sight the recipient.

The hospital administration convinced Wong to hold a press conference to relieve the strain of press, radio, and television journalists swarming the hospital. At the Institute, Li and Wong stopped all telephone calls and conferred with Zicheng in Wong's office. Wong said, "I think we should consult Mr. Moon about the press conference. I'll try to get him on the speakerphone."

Fortunately, they were able to contact Moon almost immediately. They explained the situation in Harbin and the clamor to identify and meet the transplant recipient. Zicheng had been dreading his first public exposure and had not thought it would come so soon. After listening to Wong's discussion and hearing Zicheng's reluctance, Moon suggested, "Why not have the press conference and concentrate on the surgical breakthrough? Promise the press a more detailed conference later, with an opportunity then to hear from the recipient."

With a sigh of relief from Zicheng, Wong accepted the suggestion and began preparation for the press conference later in the day. Zicheng called Lishan to join him, then slipped back to his apartment and turned on CNN China. Lishan arrived shortly after, and they watched the press conference, held mostly in English but with some of the

Chinese press receiving answers in Mandarin. The session began with an address from the hospital director, who pointed out the hospital's leading status in transplant operations. His discussion of the hospital facilities, the outstanding staff, and the diverse range of transplants done rankled Zicheng, who commented, "It sounds like a commercial for the place. Is he trying to drum up international business?"

The director described the Institute as a world leader and Dr. Wong as an eminent professor. Wong restricted his remarks to an explanation of the surgery. He did not explain the pre-operative preparation. He took several questions but, citing patient confidentiality, refused to identify either the recipient or the donor.

An insistent CNN reporter asked, "Was the donor a prisoner?"

Wong fixed him with a stony gaze and pointed to another questioner. After an hour, the administrative director declared the conference closed and thanked everyone for coming. Back in the apartment, Zicheng felt relieved but understood that a major test was in front of him.

The *Lancet* decided to publish only a few of the letters received about the transplant. With Wong and Moon's consent, Zicheng submitted the most dramatic response published by the *Lancet*:

Dear Sirs:

I write as the donor body's recipient described in the recent article by Doctors Wong and Li. A traumatic accident had left me without a lower body. There was no prospect of returning to a medical career; I planned to kill myself. The experimental surgery saved my life by restoring my existence as a person. The resumption of my surgical career was a bonus. I am grateful to the skilled team that saved my life and career. I have no regrets. I thank the Institute team. I also thank the anonymous donor in whose body I now reside.

Name withheld at writer's request.

CHAPTER 13

A few days after the press conference, Zicheng received a letter from Mr. Moon inviting him to Singapore for a meeting. The letter encouraged him to bring "your lady companion" for a four-day visit. The dates mentioned coincided with Lishan's current vacation time before the start of her residency. He assumed Wong would not object, so Zicheng accepted the invitation by email. He and Lishan could postpone their earlier travel plans.

Lishan was excited by the news. "How wonderful! I would never have imagined they would include me in the invitation. I have heard so much about Singapore. I'm dying to see it. Where will we stay?"

"We'll stay at the Four Seasons Hotel. I know that Canadian chain, and they're always excellent. And, by the way, he is sending his plane for us again."

"I've heard that Singapore is very fashion conscious. I'm glad you bought your beautiful new suit. I should probably buy another simple dress. I would not want to embarrass you."

They left a few mornings later in the familiar plane with the same pilot. A smartly uniformed female flight attendant brought Lishan a soda and Zicheng a beer. A snack tray held Latiao, duck neck, and candied fruit on a stick. She also informed them she would be serving a luncheon. There were no other passengers. During the flight, Lishan produced several pages of information she had downloaded concerning Singapore attractions.

A uniformed driver met them at the baggage claim at Singapore's Changi Airport. Stepping outside the terminal, Zicheng was disappointed at the gray air through which the sunlight forced its way. He had forgotten that Singapore ranks as one of the world's worst cities for air quality, in the same league as Harbin. The Maybach Mercedes whisked them smoothly to the hotel. The Four Seasons lobby awed Lishan. A uniformed concierge met them at the door, introduced herself in perfect English, and escorted them to a luxury suite on the fortieth floor. Their spacious suite looked out over part of the harbor and across a waterway to the science center pavilions behind a manicured soccer field. In the distance stood the iconic three-tower hotel supporting what appeared to be a full-size ship across the three rooftops.

A silver ice bucket contained a chilled bottle of champagne; beside it was a small plate of finger sandwiches. "Give me your passports. I'll check you in and then bring them back to you," said the concierge. "Feel free to have dinner in our dining room or order in-room service. To maintain your privacy, we will not divulge your registration to anyone. If there is anything I can do, please do not hesitate to call. I am at your service." She left after a slight bow.

There were three cream-colored envelopes on the bar, two for Doctor Wu Zicheng and the third addressed to Doctor Zhou Lishan. Zicheng's first envelope was from the hotel manager expressing a warm welcome. The second message was from Mr. Moon, confirming Zicheng's appointment in Moon's office the next morning at 10. Zicheng was to expect the meeting to last until late afternoon. A car would call for him at 9:45 a.m. Lishan's envelope contained a handwritten letter from the manager of the hotel's spa, indicating that Lishan had an appointment for a one-hour massage at 10 a.m. and that hair appointments and manicures were available at her pleasure. Lishan said, "I've never had treatment like this in my entire life. Are we royalty?"

"I hope we always travel this way, but no guarantees." He smiled. "We'll be able to afford this kind of hotel. I've stayed with Four Seasons before."

They elected to try the elegant dining room, where they enjoyed an incredible level of service. Zicheng enjoyed his usual Manhattan, correctly prepared. After a veritable feast, they rode upstairs and readied for bed. "Zicheng, did you notice the bathroom has a view window over the tub?" called Lishan from the other room.

"Yeah, I thought that was cool. But I can't have any distractions now. I need to sleep tonight. I suspect I have a big day tomorrow."

After room service breakfast, Zicheng left Lishan in a robe while he went off to his appointment. Moon's office was on the eighty-eighth floor of Guoco Tower, Singapore's tallest building. A well-dressed male assistant greeted Zicheng by name and ushered him into Moon's office. His corner suite commanded a magnificent harbor view. Although the office had starkly modern furniture, the interior walls had a collection of stunning Chinese art. On a small table sat two exquisite jade bowls.

"I am Winston Moon. Welcome to my office," said the stocky, elegant gentlemen of about seventy years, who entered from a side door. Offering his hand and speaking in perfect, unaccented English, he said, "Before we start, may we offer you tea or coffee or bottled water?"

"Black coffee with no sugar would be great, please," Zicheng said as he walked to the windows to admire the view. "Incredible architecture."

"We are very proud of our city," Moon said. "It is designed as a place to do business. Please have a seat." He motioned Zicheng to an upholstered chair. "I trust your flight and accommodations were satisfactory. I have been hoping to meet you for some time." Moon explained that he was in the financial business. Beyond his work line, he was interested in promoting Chinese technology, particularly in the health field. For that reason, he had funded the Transplant Institute at Harbin. He reckoned that his investment had been a scientific success by putting China at the forefront of transplant technology. "We have many achievements at the Institute, but you represent the pinnacle of our success," Moon said proudly. "The *Lancet* article has demonstrated our skill in science to the world. I would now like to ask a favor of you. If you agree, I would like to make you available tomorrow for a limited televised interview with the BBC in their studio here."

"The BBC?"

"Yes, we need to put a person to the story so that the world will understand that you are, indeed, a functioning doctor after your surgery. We cannot screen all the questions ahead of time, but we have made some questions off-limits in our negotiations with the network.

"But that will make me a public figure. People will recognize me."

"They will blur your face so no one can recognize you. We have not divulged your name to the BBC, and they will not ask. Nor will they ask any questions concerning the donor's identity or specific details about your previous training and work in the United States. I understand you have created a story to explain your American background. Please tell me that story to refresh my memory."

"When I was going through the citizenship process, the government officials approved of my possible explanation for my American accent and training. Here is the story we created. I was born in Guangdong province, but my parents left China when I was an infant. They settled in the Boston area, where they established a small but profitable business. They had what Americans call "green cards." I was raised and educated in the U.S. A few years ago, my father had a dispute with the U.S. government and faced horrendous legal bills. They decided to return home to China, and I elected to join them. That story explains my Boston-area accent."

"In your interview, you may confirm that you are a U.S. medical graduate. I suggest you tell them the approved story concerning your parents returning to China after legal problems in the U.S. They will agree not to ask about your father's business in the U.S. Your interviewer is well known and very professional. We are confident he will not employ trick questions or scare tactics. We will limit the session to twenty minutes. Will you agree to the interview?"

Remembering his promise to the Chinese authorities as conditions of his citizenship and medical license, Zicheng swallowed hard and said, "Yes, of course. I like the limitations you've mentioned. Where will they show the program?"

"As you know, the BBC is an international news service, so we assume your story will be broadcast around the world. It's entirely likely that other networks, like CNN, will pick up the story from them."

Zicheng replied, "I made a promise to go public at some point. It sounds as if this is the time, with at least some control over the interviewing environment. When and where do you need me?"

"My car will pick you up at your hotel at 9 a.m. tomorrow. You will come here to my office to meet the BBC representative, who will then take you to their studio. After the interview, they will return you here. We are not divulging your hotel, in case they should try to track you down," said Moon, who then summoned his assistant. "Call the BBC and confirm tomorrow's arrangements."

Over a light lunch in a small dining room adjoining the office, the two men continued talking. Moon was interested in Zicheng's life story before the accident. He asked about Zicheng's impression of China but commented, "You understand that China is a vast country. I hope you will travel to many areas and experience different cultures. Embrace the country as your own. We have much to offer."

After lunch, Moon signaled for the car to return Zicheng to the Four Seasons. Lishan excitedly told him about her day of pampering, then turned to Zicheng, "Tell me about your day. Was it exciting?"

"Interesting, but not that exciting. Mr. Moon is impressive, and his office is magnificent. I agreed to do something he requested."

"What request?"

"Tomorrow morning, the BBC is going to interview me for an international broadcast."

"What are you going to say?"

"It depends on the questions. There are limitations on the topics. If they ask about my background, I'll use the story about my parents leaving Boston. You remember we discussed it before."

"I know you'll do great. I'm so proud of you."

"We'll see."

Zicheng lay awake most of the night, rehearsing in his mind answers to questions he thought likely. He reminded himself that he had to be Chinese, not American. He would admit that he liked the United States but was angry at his father's treatment by U.S. authorities. He would express pleasure at being able to resume his surgical career. If he said it carefully, the interviewer would assume he had continued his surgical career at his former Chinese hospital.

If asked about his marital status, he would admit to being in a relationship. As hard as he tried, he could not think of many possible questions since the BBC had already agreed to a limited interview.

In the morning, the Maybach again delivered him to the Guoco Tower. Moon's assistant was waiting by the door to introduce him to a tall blond man, Geoffrey Lyons. After a handshake, they walked to a smaller Mercedes for the short trip to the BBC studio. "You won't need the usual television makeup," said Lyons. "We're going to blur your face during filming to protect your identity. Do we also need to disguise your voice?"

"No, I'm not worried about disguising my voice," Zicheng replied.

Lyons then took him into the studio, where he introduced him to the interviewer, Bernard Dimbilbee. "You've had an incredible experience, doctor. Have you ever done a television interview before?"

"Never."

"There's not much to it. Just look at me and take your time to answer the questions. A camera will film you from over my shoulder, but always look at my face to keep the angle consistent. It doesn't matter much because we're blurring your face anyway. Another camera will be shooting from behind you to capture my face. That clip they're putting on your shirt is your microphone. Just ignore it. Any questions?"

Zicheng shrugged and sat in the chair provided. The brightness and heat from the lights surprised him. Upon instruction, he repeated, "Testing, testing, testing one, two, three."

To start, Dimbilbee reminded the viewers of the press conference that BBC had aired ten days earlier, then played a short clip of Wong's press conference discussing the transplant. "This good doctor has kindly agreed to this interview to confirm the earlier report of his complete recovery and resumption of his surgical career. Thank you, Doctor. Let's get started."

The interview ran very much according to Zicheng's expectations. The first unanticipated question concerned the region in the United States where he had grown up. With a slight hesitation and realizing his accent might be a giveaway, he replied, "Near Boston." The only other surprise question concerned the future of this type of surgery. Zicheng spoke with enthusiasm. "This could give hope to so many people. Consider victims of ALS, amyotrophic lateral sclerosis. Their brains may function at normal levels, and yet they are doomed. If Steven Hawking had been able to have this surgery, we would still have the benefits of his innovative thinking."

Zicheng accepted the offer to watch the interview just recorded. With great relief, he could see nothing that he would change, and his face was unrecognizable. When he got into the car to return to Moon's office, he found his brow covered in sweat. He did not see Moon when he transferred from the BBC car to the Maybach, which delivered him back to the Four Seasons.

Entering his hotel room, he was greeted by a warm hug and kiss from Lishan. "How was it? Tell me all about it."

"Easier than I thought, but I'm dead tired. Let me lie down for half an hour, then let's go out and see some of the sights and have a nice dinner, and I'll tell you all about it. I have no more obligations and no more appointments."

That afternoon, they took the cable car that ran through a tall building, then above the yacht harbor to the island with its amusement park and famous aquarium. They were stunned by the beautiful fish swimming in their artfully contrived undersea settings. Returning to the hotel feeling spent, they elected in-room dining instead of finding one of the half-dozen restaurants recommended by Moon.

For their second complete day in Singapore, Moon had supplied a driver who first took them to the arboretum and then to the enormous eight-story greenhouse with its tower of flowers. Zicheng was awed. "Look, Lishan, that tower has an elevator. Let's go."

He took her hand, and they dashed to catch the elevator as the door closed. They exited seven stories up, with an aerial view of the spectacular gardens. They took a few steps to start the path spiraling down the outside of the circular tower planted solidly with orchids.

The greenhouse gardens had specimens from every continent. A topiary dragon snaked several yards through one plot. For two hours, they stepped, stopped, and stared. Lishan's phone camera shot non-stop. Neither of them had ever seen anything comparable.

As they left the greenhouse, Lishan pulled at Zicheng's arm and pointed. "Zicheng, look at that sculpture." Lishan pointed to an enormous infant, apparently floating in mid-air like a barrage balloon, with no visible support. "Such a beautiful baby. I'd like to be a mother someday."

Zicheng's throat tightened at the remark, remembering Joanne's pregnancy. He decided against a response but instead said, "I've never seen so much beauty in one place." They marveled at the enormous artificial trees, the steel trunks planted solidly with greenery almost obscuring the structure. Walkways traversed the massive branches, also made of steel heavily planted with vegetation. At the end of the afternoon, they elected to have dinner high up in the restaurant hidden within one of the park's towering manufactured trees. They agreed that neither had ever seen a park such as this.

CHAPTER 14

Zicheng and Lishan relaxed on the flight from Singapore back to Harbin with the same royal treatment on the private plane. They chatted while sipping spritzers, followed by a luncheon of Singapore noodles. Lishan said, "I have mixed feelings about next week with my family."

"I thought you were looking forward to it."

"I am, in a way. It's a small village, and I haven't lived there for the past twelve years. My parents are very old-style and don't always understand my ambition. That said, they are excited about my return. I'm not sure what to tell them about us."

"I'll let you decide on that. Most parents would be happy for their daughter to have a doctor for a boyfriend. Ready for the residency when you get back?"

"As ready as one can get. It's a good feeling to be a doctor instead of a student. I worked hard in med school; I know residency will be even tougher."

Back in their apartment, Zicheng placed a call to his parents. He told them about the interview and the exciting time he and Lishan had in Singapore. He alerted them that one or more U.S. networks might rebroadcast the BBC segment since the Harbin press conference had received international coverage.

When Lishan flew off to her family near Chengdu, Zicheng found the apartment cold and quiet without her. On the Monday following, Zicheng walked to the laboratory building at 7 a.m. As he entered, he almost collided with Li.

Li said, "Welcome back. How was Singapore? We saw your BBC interview last night."

"It was interesting. More importantly, how is Ke?"

"He died three days ago. Massive fungal infection."

"What? Why didn't you call or text me?" asked Zicheng.

"Sorry, but there was nothing you could do."

"And what about Sung? How is he taking it?"

"He was upset. He quit the program and went home yesterday. Anyway, come along. We have a meeting with Dr. Wong."

A few steps later, they entered Wong's office.

"Welcome back, Zicheng. Your interview was great. We are awash with requests for consultations. We need to revise our schedule so we can—"

Zicheng cut him off abruptly. "I'm pissed that no one called me about Ke. More importantly, how is Sung? I need to talk to him."

Wong adopted his expressionless face and serious tone. "That is not possible. Remember, when we accepted you into our program, we gave you a new name to protect your confidentiality. We did the same for Ke and Sung. We will not divulge their names to anyone, including you."

"But I should talk to Sung. He's my friend. Can I at least send him an email?"

"That is not possible. Now let's organize our workload created by your interview. Since you mentioned the surgery as a treatment for ALS, we have had inquiries from all over the world. Yesterday, five patients flew here to Harbin, trying to get on the list for the surgery. We had not thought of the ALS opportunity, so you get the credit for that. Meanwhile, we have started prepping three more patients. We intend to do one transplant per week. We need your skills, and we will start training another two surgeons. The media blitz over the past two weeks has put us behind on our surgery schedule."

"So Ke's death gets less than a minute of discussion so we can deal with the fucking schedule. Have some damned compassion! We're just part of your grand and glorious experiment."

"Restrain your anger. We were all sad to lose Ke, but we must be professional and carry on. We want to give others the success you are enjoying."

Wong handed Zicheng and Li a schedule spreadsheet. For the remainder of the day, Zicheng seethed. He was anxious to call Lishan. That evening, he called her and recited his meeting with Wong and Li.

"Those bastards have no feeling at all. I feel like quitting," he said.

"Darling, don't do anything like that. Your transplant was a success, and others will get good results in the future. Be patient until I get home. Please, don't give up on the Institute."

"It's not easy. How is it going with your folks?"

"Everything's fine, so far. We haven't had time to talk privately yet. There was a village feast to celebrate my return, and that exhausted me. Stay calm. Watch one of your Bruins games or something. I'll call later in the week."

On her single call to Zicheng during the visit, she sounded stressed but gave no details. On her return, Lishan was visibly unhappy. She explained, "I told my parents our whole story, hoping they'd be pleased."

"And?"

"It didn't work out."

"What does that mean exactly?" he asked.

"They were appalled."

"Because of what I am? Do they think I'm some kind of Frankenstein's monster?"

"I never mentioned the transplant. It's because you're a foreigner. My mother wouldn't even look at me. She hissed when she called you "Waiguo ren.""

"Maybe they just need time—"

Lishan interrupted him, "No, they even had my brother take me aside for a lecture about this foreigner. He said I should serve the needs of our people. My family is adamant against me thinking of going to the United States, even for training."

When Zicheng asked for more details, Lishan shrugged and looked morose. He knew this was not the time to pursue the topic. "This is your last weekend of freedom before residency. Can I take you shopping tomorrow?"

"Good idea. What's that American expression, retail therapy?"

The shopping trip lifted both of their spirits. At a quiet restaurant dinner, after, Zicheng said, "Next week is a big one for you. I think you're ready for it."

"I am," she said. "I'm worried about you. You won't see much of me. You don't seem very happy."

"It's the work." He reviewed the Ke experience and his frustration with the attitude of Wong and Li. "Not only did they shrug off the Ke failure, they have no concern over using prisoners for experiments. They never question the reasons for the death sentences. Wong, in particular, thinks it is none of his business. He's only concerned with more transplants."

Lishan pointed an index finger at him. "You have to stop worrying about that. Your role is to help patients who will die without implants. You can't change Chinese law."

"I guess you're right. So I'll go with the flow."

The following Monday morning, Zicheng and Lishan walked together to the hospital grounds for her to start her residency. In parting, he said, "You are the prettiest resident in the hospital."

"But you haven't seen the others yet!"

"I don't need to. I'd kiss you goodbye, but that might look unprofessional to your peers. Good luck with the residency."

"I love you. I can't kiss you in the hospital, but I appreciate your support."

That evening, an exhausted Lishan described her day. "Since I come from a distant school, I don't know any of the other thirty-two first-year surgery residents. We each got a personal room assignment for sleeping when on-call. The senior surgery resident ran our group's first meeting. He's going to shepherd us through our first year as doctors. After he welcomed us, he turned us over to the nursing supervisor.

"This woman in her late fifties was not cowed by facing a group of doctors. She explained about writing orders and behavior protocols. She handed out pagers and said, 'You may think these are old-fashioned because you have cell phones, but I don't want to be trying to contact you for an emergency when you are texting on your cell. Please wear your pager whenever you are on call.'

"Then she said, 'If a nurse pesters you to complete some paperwork, don't blame her. Do as she tells you. If you have complaints about a nurse, first speak to the head nurse on that unit. If that doesn't work, or if you wish to complain about the head nurse, then come to my office and discuss it with me.'

"After the nursing supervisor, the resident introduced a parade of professionals: head of pathology, chief pharmacist, operating room supervisor, culinary department manager, emergency room supervisor, and admitting administrator.

"Students aren't aware those people exist, but residents have to deal with all of them.

"At lunchtime, we learned about the cafeteria's queuing priorities. Orientation continued after lunch. By late afternoon, when I finally found my call room, I had information overload. Tomorrow we tour the hospital and visit our assigned units."

Zicheng listened patiently to Lishan's less-than-inspiring day. He had assumed that Harbin General Hospital would be very much like any American teaching hospital. He decided to remain silent about some of the other issues she would invariably encounter, including unwritten rules, doctors' egos, and rivalry among residents. From what he had seen in Harbin and from discussions with Li, rude behavior was even more common here than in America. He reconsidered warning her to expect sexual harassment (possibly even groping) by more senior residents and the medical staff. Lishan's focus would now switch from focusing on Zicheng to coping with the demands of the residency program.

"You don't seem very interested in my first day as a real doctor."

"I'm still upset at Wong and Li with their attitude. I'll have to get over it."

The following day, Zicheng approached the laboratory with a belligerent attitude. The first person he met was Wong, who stopped him to say, "Rumor is that the new surgeon on the transplant team is the doctor in the BBC segment. I should also warn you that the hospital staff who did not know of your surgery are now very aware. None of them should know your previous identity. You can expect a lot of stares and quite a few questions. You are now our celebrity surgeon, but within the Institute, your title is still Assistant Surgeon.

So, let's move on to the schedule for this week."

The BBC interview was a frequent topic of conversation among most of the hospital staff. Those who missed the broadcast saw the interview recorded by their friends or family. Almost everyone was proud of Dr. Wong's accomplishment. While scrubbed in for a kidney transplant, Zicheng was shocked by one of the surgeons remarking, "This is minor surgery compared to your transplant." A few nurses claimed to have seen the incision lines in his scalp. Hospital staff leaked the gossip to several reporters who now suspected he might be the body recipient. Frequent stares made Zicheng suspicious that they were discussing him. Someone obtained his cell phone number, so he had his number changed. He began to get letters from many countries, especially the United States, addressed to Doctor Wu Zicheng at the hospital. There was no gossip concerning any previous identity. After all, his medical license showed he was Wu Zicheng.

When Zicheng discussed the gossip and reporters with Wong, there was some concern. "Whoever leaked your name was not part of the Institute team," Wong said. "I suspect it was another surgeon or one of the OR nurses. Our special surgical unit has very tight security, and all of the staff down to the janitor are sworn to secrecy with a severe penalty if they violate patient confidentiality. I am concerned that at some point, someone will identify you as the former Doctor Scully. You might think about how you will deal with it if and when it happens."

"Would I be safer if I moved from Harbin?" Zicheng asked.

Wong paused for a moment, then said, "If you move away, it will take some of the attention off Harbin. We still get many inquiries about the Institute's program. If you weren't here, the media might stop searching for our most famous patient. Hard choice. You are becoming highly skilled in robotic surgery, and I would have no problem placing you at another teaching hospital well away from here. But at the moment, we need you working on our team until we can train a replacement."

"I have to think about it. I'm not anxious to move. I like working in the research environment here. If I want an academic career, do I have to get another degree?"

"There is no need to get another degree," replied Wong. "Publish a few good papers, and no one will notice that you have no academic degree."

There was a long discussion over dinner. Zicheng explained he was becoming paranoid about people staring and gossiping. Now the world beyond Harbin was involved. Lishan was well aware of Zicheng's harassment by the media. Besides the interview requests, one well-known author suggested helping Zicheng with a book, either "as told to" or "with the assistance of." She predicted a million-dollar advance. *Sixty Minutes* asked to do a segment featuring him. *Dancing with the Stars* invited him to audition. The media attention irritated Zicheng. "Lishan, I don't want to be famous. I just want the world to leave me alone with you and my career."

Looking concerned, she replied, "Unfortunately, you are already famous. There is no escaping that. Yes, it would be nice to have some privacy. Today, one of the other residents asked me, 'Are you living with the famous Doctor Wu Zicheng?' So, you see, we both get it. How can such an intelligent man bury his head in the sand? Do you not understand that everyone is curious about you? Get real." They finished the meal with glum faces.

To avoid media attention, Zicheng had stopped working in the regular hospital OR. On weekends, Zicheng and Lishan did not go out for fear of being recognized and followed. Going back and forth to work, Zicheng used a rear entrance and varied his routes to avoid sightings by reporters. Instead of going to the gym, he bought an elliptical trainer, which he crowded into their apartment office. So far, the press had not discovered his address. Lishan followed the same dodge-'em routine going back and forth to the hospital and complained about it.

Zicheng's comment about ALS lit up the internet and captured the attention of conventional media. Under pressure, the American ALS Society issued a press release warning that the surgery had never been used for ALS and would be some years in the future if it ever were perfected. The American Medical Association decried the Harbin surgery as unethical; it would never be performed in the United States. Cable news featured discussions among medical doctors and professors of philosophy. Major health insurers made clear they would not pay for this experimental surgery. Six ALS patients started GoFundMe campaigns to raise money for a trip to Harbin in hopes of having the surgery. Each site hoped to raise at least $1 million, although no one could estimate hospital and surgical costs.

Zicheng surfed the internet for the term Wu Zicheng and found two stories. A search for "brain transplant" yielded over one hundred hits, forty-three about his surgery. It was clear that the world was mistakenly calling it a brain transplant. When he mentioned that to Lishan, she commented, "You're probably the only person who can correct their thinking, to understand it's a body transplant, not a brain. Maybe you have to speak up."

Zicheng raised his eyebrows. "The BBC interview went well. Do you think if I had another interview, it would clear up the misconceptions?"

"I have no idea about that kind of thing," she answered. "I can't help you much with your new decisions. While you were a patient in the hospital, my medical and engineering know-how helped you, even if you can't remember most of what I did. I'm not sure that you believed me about sleeping with you before the transplant."

"Of course, I believed you, but my memory is still a mess."

"I love you dearly, but I can't help you much, and I need to get on to *my* problems. Your problems dominate our life. I'm getting impatient with them and, frankly, a little bored. I'm more concerned about my engineering goals and my rift with my parents."

Zicheng looked morose. "I'm sorry, Lishan. I'll try to be more understanding."

Lishan's residency put a strain on their relationship. She was now working ninety to 100 hours per week and was seldom home before 10 p.m., when she would collapse into sleep. He was sympathetic, understanding it was one of the rites of passage for an MD.

At one of their rare dinners together, Lishan made an unexpected announcement. "I do not want three more years of this crap as a surgical resident," she said heatedly. "When I finish here next June, I want to get going on my original goal to become a biomedical engineer."

Zicheng raised his eyebrows. "And how would you do that?"

"With my medical credentials, I can probably get an engineering job with one of the companies doing advanced research and product development. And get paid!" She looked almost defiant as she stared at Zicheng.

"Here or in the States?"

"I don't know. Probably here in China. We're as good or better in our science, and I wouldn't have to go through your immigration hassle. I have to start searching on the internet to see what is available."

"Can I help?" he asked. He heard Lishan's frustration and noted her reference to staying in China. *Where was this coming from?* "A few months ago, you were interested in finishing your residency in the States. Have you changed your mind?"

"I have a lot of doubts about it. I don't want more residency training anywhere, so that's changed. I also think we should stay in China."

Because of their earlier discussions, he had assumed that Lishan would willingly move to the U.S. if that were his eventual choice. This was something different. He repeated, "Is there anything I can do to help?"

"Not at the moment. When I get more clarity, we'll talk about it."

Late one evening, Zicheng's father called. When they connected, Walter said, "We watched you on BBC last night. That was exciting. You did a great interview. The only surprise was that you admitted you had grown up near Boston."

"I was afraid my accent would give me away. And in this kind of situation, you should tell as few lies as possible. I found out that the press now knows my Chinese name. The *Wall Street Journal* even has an American reporter fluent in Mandarin staked out at the hospital. It's not fun."

"Why don't you come home to Natick?" his father suggested.

"That wouldn't solve anything. Running away is not the answer." He expressed his concern about the confusion between brain and body transplants. He suggested he might put the misunderstanding to rest and end the publicity by having another interview. Roger asked for his father's opinion.

"I think you don't understand. The public is not interested in the terminology. People are fascinated by the idea that a person can live on in another body. Your comment about Steven Hawking was a lightning bolt. You underestimate your importance and influence."

His father continued, "You remember my cousin Bill Wright? He's had a good career in public relations. I trust him. What if I give him a call, explain the situation, and get his advice?"

"I think that's a good idea. I need help in thinking this through. Is Mom there?" His mother got on the screen.

"I was so proud to see you on television. You did so well!"

Roger assured his parents that he would not make any public statements until he heard from Bill Wright.

The next Monday, Wong asked Zicheng if he had any further thoughts or had decided about moving. "I'd rather not move," answered Zicheng. "I have to think for the long term and not settle for a short-term solution that might be wrong in the end. I'll certainly be here until you can get a replacement." Zicheng understood that he was making a commitment of at least six months to a year. He scrubbed in and executed a delicate robotic operation on a dog but found himself distracted by thoughts of his future. He went home scowling, angry at weaving a different route every evening to avoid reporters.

Since their success with Zicheng, despite Ke's death, Wong and his team had done two more successful corporeal transplants, all now in the recovery phase. From that experience, Wong and Li concluded this was now an accepted treatment rather than a surgical experiment. Zicheng felt some encouragement over the successes but retained concerns over the donor sourcing. The hospital administrator was interested in expanding his facility to provide Wong and his team with more operating rooms and beds. At least one foreign investment group with a Chinese partner had visited Harbin for discussions with both the hospital and Wong concerning the possibility of opening a freestanding for-profit transplant hospital. The Chinese central government sent a senior official to Harbin to monitor the situation.

Zicheng did not participate in any negotiations, nor was he a key decision-maker. He enjoyed the surgery but most of all, he found satisfaction in guiding the patients through recovery, which he remembered so well. However, he felt he was living in a whirlwind. The time pressures made it more and more challenging to concentrate on his work. Without warning to Zicheng, two neurosurgeons suddenly appeared at the Institute for robotic training. Li instructed Zicheng to train them as quickly as possible for an anticipated rush of patients.

Zicheng was surprised at the speed with which changes were happening. Suddenly, a contracting company was on-site, constructing a significant new building for the Institute's clinical activities. Three new transplant candidates now occupied the cottage.

Off the hospital grounds, but nearby, another structure was rising, surrounded by a prison-like fence topped with barbed wire. Li explained to Zicheng, "That's our donor dormitory; some people call it The Farm. Potential donor prisoners work in a large vegetable garden while awaiting the call to their final surgery." From a series of sheds and pens, they heard the cackle of hens, the honking of geese, and grunts of hogs. Zicheng pondered the irony of The Farm, whose main function was harvesting organs for transplant, not producing food for the hospital. Each day, passing The Farm en route to the hospital or back, Zicheng felt revulsion at what the stockade represented.

Zicheng now worked at least sixty hours a week. The Institute was doing three body-brain transplants per week. Each transplant operation took an average of fifteen hours. Zicheng requisitioned two sets of elastic stockings to avoid venous stasis from standing for long periods. He was disappointed that he had no say in patient selection, scheduling, or team assignments.

Zicheng finally received an email from Bill, the public relations expert, who said that while he was not competent to advise Roger, he had the name of an appropriate consultant in Beijing who might help. Wilfrid Chung was Chinese-born and Ivy League-educated. He spent several years with Ogilvy and Mather in the U.S. before returning to China to start his own business. Although he specialized in assisting U.S. companies in functioning in China, Chung had healthcare experience in the United States. zicheng was immediately interested and sent off an email to Chung. After a quick exchange of emails, they agreed to meet in Beijing.

Lishan continued to work 100 or more hours per week, with only occasional nights at home in the apartment. Between her exhaustion and Zicheng's tiredness, lovemaking was becoming sporadic and less satisfying. Zicheng was still receiving a barrage of offers from abroad, one of which appeared tempting. The American Society of Transplant Surgeons invited Dr. Wu Zicheng to address a plenary session at their annual meeting in Bal Harbor, Florida, in January. They asked him to speak on "Corporeal Transplant: Patient and Surgeon Perspectives." The Society would pay all travel expenses and an honorarium of $10,000.

The evening the offer arrived, Lishan was home for dinner and off-call. "Lishan, I am tempted by this speaking offer," he said. "I think there needs to be a full explanation of the surgery procedure and a frank discussion about the use of prisoners as organ donors. After I talk to Wilfrid Chung in Beijing, we'll decide on the Florida offer."

She paused. "You say, 'we'll decide.' You mean that 'you'll decide.' I'm not part of the decision. You'll do as you please." She shook her head and glared.

"What's wrong now?"

"Going to Florida will make you a celebrity, so you've decided on that issue. It looks to me like you're going back to the States permanently."

"We still haven't decided on that. We're still looking into the question of your immigration status if we moved back."

"You keep saying, 'if we moved **back**,' when I've never been there. I've never agreed to go to America. I'm not ruling it out, but don't make assumptions."

They ended the conversation with Zicheng puzzled. *What had gone wrong?*

Two days later, Zicheng flew to Beijing. He did not ask permission for the day off. After considerable thought, he had decided to share his accurate history with Wilfred Chung. He had also concluded that his story would become public if he returned to the U.S. With nothing scheduled in the OR, he could skip training the neurosurgeons, whom he now viewed as his replacements. His morning flight to Beijing placed him in Chung's public relations office shortly before noon. Over lunch at Chung's club, Roger first told the story of his medical odyssey. He then explained his current predicament. "Wu Zicheng is now a public figure; Roger Scully is on no one's radar. And I'm unhappy with my Institute status, which is unlikely to improve."

"Do you want to move back to the States?" asked Chung.

"Right now, I would like nothing more than to live in the good old USA. Unfortunately, I am a Chinese man with a made-up history and an American man with a secret name and buried background. All that is confusing to deal with and very difficult to explain."

"I can understand your confusion."

"I'm also concerned about Zhou Lishan. We've discussed a future together, but as yet, we've made no plans. U.S. immigration disapproves of Americans taking foreign spouses. U.S. consular officials are not allowed to perform marriages. So, any marriage in China would be between two Chinese citizens, and Roger Scully does not exist as a Chinese citizen. It's complicated but important in my decision-making. For Lishan to apply for admission to a U.S. medical residency will be horrendously difficult. She now is thinking of looking for an engineering job."

"I'm sorry I can't help you on the relationship issue," said Chung. "I can refer you to a good U.S. immigration lawyer here in Beijing. I'm sure she's dealt with similar problems before."

"You're right. I should get legal advice about Lishan's immigration."

"Let's discuss your status as a celebrity. You've been through physical and psychological hell, with incredible amounts of pain and suffering. Consider those as dues you have paid. You have every right to monetize that experience. You're a person of sterling character with a compelling personal story. Through no fault of your own, that story will create controversy over the ethics of the procedure. Be careful not to get tarred with the ethics brush. At no time did you do anything even remotely wrong or suspicious. I think we can help you preserve your image."

"My image is in danger?" Zicheng asked.

"Certainly. Some people will try to exploit your experience as a reason to criticize China's policies and practices. You must never admit to doing something unethical by accepting your transplant." Leung looked very serious.

"I have an immediate decision to make," Zicheng told Chung. "I have an invitation to address the American Society of Transplant Surgeons in Bal Harbor, Florida. It's a prestigious event, and I would be a featured speaker. What do you think?"

"That sounds like a great way for Doctor Roger Scully to go public. If you're comfortable with finally allowing the world to see the connection between Doctor Scully and Doctor Wu, then this is your opportunity. If you want to preserve the gap between those two people, I advise against the speaking engagement. Where do you stand on preserving the distinction?" asked Chung.

"Sooner or later, probably sooner, someone from outside the Institute will find out my secret. The world will find out that Wu Zicheng was Roger Scully. The speaking engagement is still four months away, so we have time to work out some of the details. What else would you suggest?"

Chung paused to think. "You need an agent. That sounds crass and commercial, but a good agent will help you in several ways. They will negotiate contracts much better than you are likely to do. The agent can help you with scheduling, including travel. That person can also protect you from much of the harassment by the media."

"I never thought of an agent, but it would give me a buffer from the requests I've been getting, including things as wild as *Dancing with the Stars*."

Chung smiled and continued, "I'll give you the names and contact information for two of my U.S. colleagues. Both are reliable, ethical, and expensive. I understand your dissatisfaction with the Institute, but be very careful not to piss off your boss. Not only can the Institute fire you, but they can make your life hell if they complain to the Chinese government. Understand that you are and always will be, *waiguo ren*, and not to be fully trusted. Have you heard that expression before?"

"Someone said it about me but never to me."

"It's a slang expression for a foreigner, usually used in a derogatory sense. By now, you should understand that China is the most xenophobic nation on earth. You will never be fully accepted here, despite your citizenship, appearance, and manufactured history."

"Okay," Roger acknowledged. "I'll be a good laborer and keep my mouth shut. I'll also speed up my plans to get out of here. When you're back in your office, please text me the contacts for the immigration attorney and the two American agents. I also need to arrange payment for you. What are your terms?"

"Your situation is unique. I usually represent large corporations with ongoing issues. From them, I ask for a retainer of $10,000 U.S. dollars. For you, if you give me a check for $2,000, that will cover today and any further minor questions."

"No problem," Roger said, pulling out his checkbook.

The two American agents recommended by Chung responded almost immediately to Roger's emails. Since he was concerned about possible government monitoring of his email, he suggested interviews via WeChat. Both agents were personable and asked similar questions. When one appeared to be pushing to manage his investments, he selected the other, Lois Marshall. She addressed him as Dr. Scully. He did not mention a possible move back to the U.S. He promised to email her a complete CV and a narrative of his time in China. She would send him her standard contract via email.

A few days later, Zicheng had his regular monthly appointment with Doctor Chu, the immunologist. "We are pleased with your progress, rejection-wise," she said. "The drug you take is part-way through the American FDA approval. We plan to market it in America. Our clinical trials here were acceptable in quality for the FDA, but they still insist on a larger American trial, which is now underway. If that works as well as we think, we should get FDA approval early next year. Let's keep you on your current dose, which is pretty low, for another three months, and then check your blood work." Zicheng was relieved, thinking he could stay on the same medications if and when he moved back to the States. He shared the news with Lishan the same evening.

"My immune system is stable. Amy Chu says the U.S. FDA is about to approve her drug."

"Is that important?"

"I'm probably on it for life, and with American approval, it means I would have no problem in getting my prescriptions there."

Lishan explained, "We still need to talk about *my* future. You're solving your questions about a return to the States. We still haven't decided what I'm doing. You promised you would look into the immigration question."

"I'll get on to that right away. I have an immigration attorney referral."

To address Lishan's concerns, Zicheng contacted Ms. Mai Ling, the Beijing immigration attorney. She responded, suggesting a telephone call. Ling said there would be no charge for the initial call, but if he retained her to work on his behalf, she required a deposit of $5,000 in U.S. dollars. When they connected by telephone, Zicheng first gave his abbreviated medical history. He then explained about his likely return to the United States and his relationship with Lishan. Though they hadn't yet made plans to marry, if they decided to do so, he asked Ling if they should take that step in China or the U.S. What were Lishan's immigration options, either way? What were the steps needed for her to obtain a medical residency in the U. S.? Ling agreed to be retained upon receipt of his check and estimated it would be two to four weeks before she could get answers from U.S. officials. Ms. Ling addressed him as Doctor Wu Zicheng.

At the Institute, the team was preparing three potential body recipients, all white males. One was from South Africa, one from Australia, and one from the United States. The Institute regularly accepted foreign patients, despite the Chinese law prohibiting "medical tourism" for transplants. To quell international outrage, the government had announced the prohibition but applied no enforcement at the local level, where transplant tourism was profitable.

The American and South African candidates both had ALS. It was clear that all three were willing to change their race. Zicheng noticed that the next group of three on the schedule were all white females. Zicheng asked Li, "I notice we are now going to be offering corporeal transplants to women. Do many women in China get capital punishment?"

"Ah, they are probably all Muslim Uyghurs who get into a lot of trouble," Li answered. "Some might be followers of Falun Gong, that crazy religious group. I don't think we'll have any shortage of donors." Though Zicheng said nothing, he was startled at how easily Li referred to having a supply of donors among women from a religious minority. *Is this an abuse of the system to create more donors? Should I be killing these women when I remove their brains? I'd feel better doing a kidney transplant where both the donor and recipient live on, but brains are different. What might happen if the U.S. started using prisoner donors, at least for kidneys?*

CHAPTER 15

Zicheng continued to work sixty-hour weeks without complaint. Wong and Li were pleased with his training of the two neurosurgeons. For his part, Zicheng displayed a positive attitude with no indication that he might leave Harbin. The Institute schedule showed one week with no surgery. On inquiry, he found that Wong and Li would be in Beijing for a medical conference in the first week of September. He had an idea that he raised that evening with Lishan. "If I can get two weeks off early next month, I'd like to do that trek in Tibet that I missed due to the accident. Can you get time off?"

"No way. They made it clear that there are no vacations in the first six months, and even funerals would only be two days off. If you can go, that's fine. You need a break, and it's something you have always wanted to do. Go for it." From the tone of her response, Roger surmised that Lishan had no interest in trekking. Without further discussion, Zicheng decided to postpone any Tibetan adventure.

"Well, could you at least get two days off and go with me to Chengdu? I'd like to see Dr. Wen and his team to thank them for saving my life. I'm sure they will be curious and happy to see what I look like now. They only remember me as the half-person they created with the hemicorporectomy. That was an amazing feat of surgery."

She brightened at the mention of Chengdu, her medical school. "That sounds doable. I can also see a few of my classmates." They immediately consulted her schedule and found the appropriate days. The next morning, he called Dr. Wen. "Remember me? You saved my life when I was Dr. Roger Scully; you sent me to Harbin. I am now Doctor Wu Zicheng, working at the Harbin Institute as a surgeon. I'd like to have a visit with you."

Wen replied, "I was aware that the surgery was a success but have heard nothing since. I would love to see you. When we heard about the transplant and saw the BBC interview, I guessed it might be you. When could you come here?"

"That's why I am calling," Zicheng said. "I am coming to Chengdu the week after next. Could we have dinner while I am there? You choose the restaurant. Your former student, Zhou Lishan, will be with me. Bring the whole team that helped me."

"Would you be so kind as to do surgical grand rounds while you are here? I would love for the residents and everyone else to hear about your transplant. I still have pictures of you before and after the hemicorporectomy."

"I would be glad to do that. After all, you saved my life. If you're going to use pictures of me, can you avoid showing the face? Most people don't know I was formerly a white man."

"Of course. My team remembers you, but there is no reason to publicize your race."

Zicheng and Wen set a time and place for dinner. Zicheng and Lishan would arrive on Thursday to dine that night with Wen and his team. Zicheng would present at rounds the following morning; Lishan arranged a Friday dinner with some of her medical class friends. They would be in Chengdu for two nights. He would clear the time with Wong and Li.

"Li, I'm tired and need a break. We have nothing important scheduled for next week. Can I have a vacation?"

"You know Wong and I will be away, so it's no problem. We owe you some time off, anyway. Are you going out of town?"

"I'm going to Chengdu for two days, plus I have a lot of personal things to do right here, like getting my driver's license. I'll be available if you need me for anything urgent."

"Right, then, I'll take you off the schedule that week."

On the first vacation day, Zicheng went to the government office to obtain a driver's manual and a learner permit. He was not looking forward to city driving; Harbin traffic was mad chaos in a wretched atmosphere of smoke and exhaust. He hoped driving in the countryside would be more pleasant. Adjacent to the permit office was a driving school, where he arranged for lessons to begin the following day.

Determined to see some of the few Harbin tourist attractions, he took a taxi to the Daowai Mosque, the largest mosque in Harbin, erected in 1897. As he strolled around the square in front of the mosque, he was aware of the heavy police presence, including several persons he reckoned were plainclothes police officers. The familiar surveillance cameras seemed everywhere. For once, he found his ever-present facemask reassuring. It protected him not only from the foul air but also disguised his face from those cameras. As he raised his phone to photograph the mosque, he heard shouting. Two plainclothes policemen were dragging a young man toward a waiting police van. Zicheng quickly put his phone in his pocket and turned to leave the square. He wanted no part of police action, especially where they were grabbing a Uyghur.

Suddenly, a heavy hand on his shoulder spun him around. He

stared into the face of a scowling policeman. Two more were running toward him. While the first cop zip-tied his hands behind his back, another went into his pocket for the cellphone. Another hand reached into his coat and retrieved his wallet. No one was speaking to him.

In Mandarin, Zicheng asked, "What is going on?"

"You are coming with us, Uyghur hoodlum." was the reply as a police van drove up.

Loudly, Zicheng replied that he was not Uyghur. They ignored him. Within seconds, they threw him roughly into the back of the van, as he protested in Mandarin, "Not Uyghur, not Uyghur!" As he landed in the body of the van, his skull hit the bench with a thud. His head began to ache as fireworks erupted in his brain. He lay on the floor, in a fetal position, for the ten-minute ride.

At the police station, two officers yanked him from the van and took him inside. At the counter near the entrance stood a camera at face level. They pushed him into place to take his picture with and without his mask. The police unfastened his wrists and placed his hands, palms down, onto a transparent screen built into the counter. *Instant mug shot and fingerprints*, he realized. While Zicheng continued protesting, three men hustled him into a small interrogation room. From the desk he had just left, he heard a shout. The desk officers had found a match for his face from the computer system. Zicheng was feeling his bruised temple as they pushed him against the wall. No wet blood, but his skin was starting to swell, and fireworks continued in his brain. Someone spun him around to put his back to the concrete block wall. The man pushing him reached for Zicheng's belt and released the buckle. Without undoing buttons or zipper, he yanked down Zicheng's trousers and then jockey shorts. With a wide grin, the cop stood back and pointed to Zicheng's penis. "See, Uyghur." The circumcision had confirmed their suspicion.

Zicheng grimaced with pain from his bruised head. The ringing headache brought back memories of his surgery recovery period. He mentally composed his Mandarin words, then spoke up, "I want a lawyer. Right now."

One of the desk officers had just entered, in time to hear Zicheng's request. He responded, "Uyghurs don't need lawyers. They need to behave themselves." The four policemen stood for several minutes, ignoring Zicheng while congratulating themselves and making rude comments, many concerning Zicheng's penis size. They brought in a female police officer to view the spectacle. She covered her smile with her hand.

Zicheng reddened with anger and frustration. *How the fuck did this happen? Now, what'll they do with me?*

Suddenly, a more senior officer strode in and snarled at the group. "Fools! You arrested Doctor Wu Zicheng. We saw him on the BBC program about the Harbin brain transplant. When you found his face and fingerprints on the computer match, you should have read the text and realized it was a match for an executed prisoner. Doctor Wu has that body, but he's not a Uyghur." The policewoman and two of the officers fled the room.

Zicheng had listened with amazement as he pulled up his trousers with his freed hands.

The senior officer spoke again, this time in perfect English. "Doctor Wu, I apologize for your treatment, but we must be careful with Uyghurs and their sympathizers. My car will take you back to your home or hospital or anywhere in the city. Your social profile confirms you were the recipient of the transplant. We will not bother you again, but please understand that the law prohibits anyone from taking photographs or videos of police actions." The junior officer handed Zicheng his phone, wallet, passport, and keys.

The senior officer asked, "Would you like some water?"

"No, just take me home," Zicheng said.

Zicheng gave the officer's driver directions to his apartment. Once there, he examined his scalp in the mirror. No broken skin, but an egg-size bump was swelling. Somewhat light-headed, he made his way to the refrigerator and pulled out a bag of frozen peas, which he applied to his bruise. Then he sat down and called Lishan. Not surprisingly, he got her voice mail. "Lishan, call me ASAP. I'm home after getting beaten by some cops."

Lishan called within five minutes. "Zicheng, what has happened to you? Are you hurt?"

Zicheng explained the circumstances of his detention and then moved on to discuss the medical implications. "They rang my bell when I hit my head on a bench. I wasn't unconscious at any time, but I have a nasty swelling. I don't need any treatment except for ice packs and Tylenol."

"I'm coming right home. Don't move until I get there in ten minutes."

Lishan arrived, looking anxious and hurried. Rushing to Zicheng, she gently parted his hair to get a better look. "It's like you said it was. Your swelling is just below the suture line from your operation, but everything seems intact. Let me look at your pupils."

She pulled a penlight from her breast pocket. With a serious face and steady gaze, she examined his eyes. "Pupils equal and reactive, so that's good. Do you think we should go to the ER and get an x-ray?"

"No, but I'd feel better if you could stay home for a few hours."

"Of course, I've already arranged that. Have you had any Tylenol yet?"

"No, but you can get me a few."

When he took the pills and tried to take some water, his hands shook so that Lishan helped steady the glass. He kicked off his shoes and laid on the bed, the bag of peas next to his temple. By evening, he reported only a slight headache.

Lishan reheated a take-out dinner of fried dumplings. They picked at small portions.

"Now, I know how a Uyghur feels. They get treated like shit."

"I'm sorry it happened to you. The police treated you horribly. The cops misbehaved, but try to understand that when Uyghurs make a lot of trouble, they make bad blood with the police."

"I'm not sure that explains all their actions. I forgot to tell you, the senior police officer spoke to me in *English*, if you can imagine. I'm sure that when he went into the computer system, he found out the relationship of Wu Zicheng to Roger Scully. I find that scary."

"I suspect it's your social profile, but authorities restrict access to the profile information."

"What the hell is a social profile?"

"We have a social credit scoring system. I have heard that the U.S. has a credit score system for financial information. China goes further and scores financial and non-financial information, including data from the facial recognition system. If you are doing something patriotic, then it will show up. If you are doing something bad, like protesting against the government, then it will show up as well."

"Can I see my social profile?"

"I don't think so, but I've never known anyone to ask for their profile. Everyone knows about the social profile system. Are you going to bed now?'

"That sounds like a good idea. Are you home for the night?"

"Yes, and I'll check on you every two hours until I get up at six. I wish I could kiss it better for you."

"I appreciate that. You're always there for me."

The next morning, Zicheng took two Tylenol for his slight

headache, canceled his driving lesson, and headed for the familiar shopping mall. On the way, he reviewed his relationship with Lishan. He had not appreciated her dedication to him. At the mall, his first stop was a jewelry store, where he made a purchase.

After that, while shopping for a better audio system for their apartment, he passed a window filled with musical instruments, including guitars. His memory flashed back to his medical school amateur band, the Rockin' Docs, where he played acoustic guitar. With some trepidation, he entered the store. Wondering if his fingers would still work and play chords, he shrugged and picked up a guitar. There was no familiar feel to the neck and strings. He realized he would have to relearn his previous skills. With pursed lips, he compared instruments before selecting an American-made Gibson, a familiar brand. He completed his purchase with a case and an English language instruction book titled *Beginning Guitar*. He hurried back to the apartment, anxious to regain the musical part of his identity. *I'm going to have some fun for a change*, he thought as he anticipated playing music. He texted Lishan that they would dine that night at their favorite restaurant.

After they were seated, Zicheng reassured Lishan of his lack of headache or other symptoms. She returned to the events of the previous day. "I can't believe what happened to you yesterday. I'm sorry—"

He held up his hand. "Lishan, it's not your fault. Let's just agree that the Chinese government does not treat Uyghurs properly. I'm fine and wasn't badly hurt. It's a bit scary that my social profile, as they call it, identifies me as being an organ recipient. But then, in this country, the government knows everything. Let's change the subject."

With that, they turned to the menus and discussed their choices among the duck entrees. When they had ordered the food, he smiled at her. "Oh, another thing, my dearest Lishan," he said, leaning across the table to kiss her. "I have a surprise for you." He retrieved a small box from his pocket and opened the lid. "In Ireland, this is called a promise ring. I give it to you as a token of my love, in appreciation for your steadfast care during the most difficult periods of my life." She smiled as he placed the mosaic of gems on her left ring finger. Her face radiated a surge of love toward this man with whom she had become so close.

"That's so sweet of you to give me such a precious gift," she said. "I love you, too. I have never heard of a promise ring. I love it, but perhaps you could explain it. I assume it's not the same as an engagement ring."

"Let's say it's close to an engagement ring. It represents our deep love for each other. We decided before that we weren't yet ready for marriage. We've had uncertainties about my citizenship, my future, and your career. We're making some progress, at least concerning my status. Let's talk about our future."

Lishan said, "We've been preoccupied with your status, which was appropriate. But we still have not had a serious conversation about *my* career."

He poured them each a glass of wine, and they reached toward each other to hold hands. "I must admit I haven't paid enough attention to your career ideas. I have the immigration attorney looking into what's involved in you moving to the States, so I have been thinking of you."

With a frown, she said, "You didn't tell me you were seeing an immigration attorney."

"By giving you the promise ring, I want to acknowledge how my love for you has grown since we first met. You not only cared for my physical needs but gave me the hope and encouragement I needed to survive. I was so lonely and isolated."

"I remember those days. You were in bad shape."

"When you moved into the cottage with me, you couldn't have given me any greater gift. You counseled me when I was deciding to accept the body transplant. And when you said you loved me, that was frosting on the cake." He squeezed her hands.

Zicheng continued, "When we moved into the apartment, we were both so happy. We talked about a future life together and what that would mean."

"That was one of my happiest days."

"We didn't anticipate the complications since. My PTSD has been a problem, but the medication is helping. Ever since the *Lancet* article, you've seemed more and more distant. Do I imagine things? What going on?"

Lishan looked down, withdrew her hands from his, and folded them in front of her. "Please be patient while I think this through," she asked. Then, in a slow and soft voice, she said, "When I first saw you, I was overwhelmed with pity. I could not imagine how you could live with half a body; I wanted to do anything I could. I was thrilled when the chariot made such a difference in your life. I admit, there was an element of pride in me to be the student chosen to tend to this disfigured foreigner."

"Your chariot invention was incredible."

"As we became acquainted, I admired your persistence and energy. I grew to think of myself as your best friend. I was glad to come to Harbin with you because I didn't want you to face such mind-boggling surgery alone. Sleeping with you in the cottage helped me, too, because I enjoyed your close touch."

Zicheng nodded, "You were with me when I wasn't good for anything."

"After you had a complete body, I felt our friendship move to something else. I felt loved and needed when you suggested this apartment. With your apprenticeship and your Chinese citizenship, I saw us living out our lives in China."

"I thought we might do that." He nodded.

Lishan continued, "Now everything has changed. You sound more like you intend to go back to the States. You spend all your time reading American newspapers and watching American TV. I don't like the chaos that has erupted over the story of your transplant. There is no way you can avoid worldwide attention. That'll inevitably channel your life away from China. So I have to deal with that and decide what I want for my own life."

Zicheng reached for her hands again and said, "But I've already inquired about immigration for you and asked about getting you a residency in the United States. You know I want you to come with me."

"Yes, I know that's what you've said. But I'm not sure that's what's best for me. We've never discussed whether you would stay in China to follow *my* career."

"I have to admit that I haven't given that much thought," he said.

"Neither of us like Harbin. As I asked before, would you move to another province for my career?" Lishan inquired.

"That's a tough question. I have to admit I'm not always comfortable living in China."

They sat quietly for a few minutes. Lishan broke the silence by saying, "Why don't we continue to think about it? I need to pack for tomorrow's trip. Let's go home."

Back at the apartment, she quickly retreated into the bedroom, packed silently, and was in bed within minutes. They were leaving the next day for Chengdu, and both welcomed a change of scene.

When they arrived in Chengdu, Zicheng smiled at the balmy 65F temperature. The bitter cold of Harbin suffered in comparison. From their hotel, they taxied to the restaurant Cheng Du, considered Chengdu's finest. The restaurant was cavernous in size. Zicheng's face brightened when he smelled the sweet and spicy peppers for which the region is famous. When they spotted Wen at a round table with four other men, Zicheng walked over, offered his hand, and, in perfect Mandarin, said, "Good evening, Dr. Wen. I am Dr. Wu Zicheng, also known as Roger Scully. And I am sure you remember Dr. Zhou Lishan, who was one of your students."

As they shook hands, Dr. Wen stared wide-eyed at Zicheng's face. "Incredible," he said. "I never would have thought it possible. You may or may not remember these men, your original treatment team." He then proceeded to introduce each of them. Zicheng recognized three of the four. Over drinks, they insisted he tell them everything about his treatment at the Harbin Institute. They expressed envy when he described the Harbin OR, with its micro-MRI and dual robotic consoles. Throughout the meal, the six surgeons talked shop continually. One of the junior surgeons nudged the one next to him and pointed to Zicheng, using chopsticks with obvious dexterity to maneuver some spicy chicken. They both nodded.

The surgical team joked about Roger surviving in the cold climate of Harbin, eating what they called "Russian stews." Zicheng felt warmed to be treated as an equal among his peers for the first time in a year. He also enjoyed being called Roger, the name which the Chengdu team remembered.

Lishan was mostly silent during the evening and looked less than happy at being ignored by the group. The next morning, she was a spectator in the audience for grand rounds. Zicheng spoke Mandarin for his presentation. The audience gasped at the pictures of his naked lower body before and after the hemicorporectomy. At the end of the appointed hour, a group of at least twenty medical staff and residents bombarded him with more questions. Zicheng was the star of Chengdu surgery.

Lishan was looking forward to dinner that night. She said, "You'll remember two of my classmates because they helped you with your first Mandarin lessons."

"Lishan, I'm sorry that I can't recall that much about that period. I'm sure you're right, but remember, I couldn't even recall the chariot until you showed me the picture."

"Well, they'll be impressed tonight when you speak Mandarin so well."

Lishan's six classmates, all of whom had remained in Chengdu as interns, greeted her with enthusiasm. Most of their interest, however, centered on Zicheng. One of them had heard his presentation at rounds and was recounting the experience to two others. A young woman approached Zicheng and asked, "Do you remember me teaching you your numbers in Mandarin? You look very different now."

"Thank you for teaching me the numbers. I do remember the lessons, but I can't remember you. Understand that my brain has been through a lot."

Throughout the dinner, most of the conversation centered on Zicheng. Only two of Lishan's classmates inquired about her residency experiences. In the taxi back to the hotel, Zicheng commented, "I'm beat. I have never answered so many questions in a day. Are your classmates doing okay?"

"They didn't say much. I feel like the ignored partner of a famous person. An appendage." Lishan fell silent. Her silence continued when they returned to their hotel and on their return flight to Harbin. Zicheng hardly noticed; he was already thinking and making notes about the op-ed he would write for the *New York Times*. Lois Marshall had strongly suggested this as a way to amplify his talk to the Bal Harbor meeting.

Back at their apartment, Lishan opened her email to find a

response from a Xinhua recruiting firm. They were enthusiastic about her credentials and saw no difficulty in placing her with one of the many bioengineering firms. They quoted a salary range far beyond her expectations. She printed out the letter and, without a word, handed it to Zicheng.

"So, you're serious about staying in China?" he asked.

Lishan frowned, "Very serious. I went to med school to become a biomedical engineer, not a practicing doctor. I've never lost that ambition. I know I can succeed here. Going to America scares me professionally and culturally. We've never discussed marriage and children. What would happen if my career was somewhere you didn't like? As I asked you before, would you follow me for *my* career?"

With raised eyebrows, Lishan responded, "Wow, those are a lot of serious questions. Marriage first, I want to marry you. That's clear in my mind. Children? I'm getting older and would like to have my children soon. I don't want them going off to college when I'm retired."

"I haven't heard that before. It sounds like you want children in the next few years."

"That's right. Wouldn't you?" Lishan asked, "If we get married, I would like children soon. But where are we going to live?"

"I can live almost anywhere in the States with my specialty. There's a doctor shortage everywhere." He raised his eyebrows as if to declare, "See, I've answered all your questions."

"You answer my questions so easily. I wonder if you are paying attention. I'm skeptical about a career for me in the U.S. When I asked, 'Would you follow me for my career,' I was asking if you would stay in China for my career," Lishan said.

Zicheng sighed and put his head in his hands, blowing softly. "I have thought about that. To be truthful, I cannot stay in China. I'm sorry if that sounds selfish, but it's true."

"Was this conclusion from your beating by the police?"

"That solidified my thinking, but I had more or less decided against China already."

"Despite how much we love each other, I worry that the marriage would not make it. You're tied to your country. I'm tied to my family. I want children, but I want them to enjoy and appreciate Chinese culture. I have nothing against American values, but they're different than ours."

"I'm shocked. I've been assuming we would marry and move home to the States and live happily ever after. My dreams just got shattered." Zicheng frowned.

"I'm sorry about that, but it's one of our differences. You always assume you have the answers, and that's the way the world will go. It's probably my fault we didn't have this discussion earlier before you built your dream life,' said Lishan.

"I think I've messed things up. Our future is looking a bit shaky, but don't write it off. Let's hope we can come up with a solution."

They stood up and hugged each other tightly. Both were crying.

Lying in bed, he had mixed feelings. Tonight, he had finally decided to move back to the USA, even if it meant losing Lishan. He had not thought of that before in trying to choose where to live. He concluded that Lishan had decided for both of them—her country and career over love. He should now plan his departure.

CHAPTER 16

For the next few months, Zicheng and Lishan had a friendly but strained relationship. Both found distraction in their work. Their sex was less frequent but still filled with passion. Twice, he found her sobbing in the bedroom. Meanwhile, a steady stream of interview requests arrived addressed to Dr. Wu Zicheng at the hospital in Harbin. He sent all invitations on to agent Lois Marshall to answer. Her usual response was, "Contact us later, in January, when the doctor might be available in the U.S." It was now late November, and Zicheng had promised to deliver a manuscript of his talk to the American Society of Transplant Surgeons by December 15.

Once he accepted the Society's invitation, Zicheng became preoccupied with the talk preparation. The surgical audience would be most interested in techniques. He was more interested in bringing to light solutions to the American problem of donor organ shortage. Every day, in the United States, seventeen people die awaiting a transplant; his Chinese experience had convinced him that reliance on capital punishment was not the solution, but the need for the transplants compelled him to offer an alternative. Giving prisoners the right to donate a kidney or liver lobe would ease and possibly obliterate the organ shortage.

Remembering his lessons from high school English, he decided to start with an outline. He put down the following:

Personal background (education, residency, ER experience)

Crush injury and surgical result (with picture)

My transplant and complications

Apprenticeship and surgical experience in China

Surgery in China

U.S. transplant situation

NYTimes op-ed

Using the outline facilitated writing the manuscript. Zicheng simply recounted the facts and allowed one paragraph for each topic, but he included the entire *New York Times* op-ed piece. He would present slides with maps of China and Tibet to show Chengdu, Harbin, and Xining. He decided to speak from a series of flashcards for his presentation but then read word-for-word the *New York Times* article. After the op-ed, he would plead to the audience to enact political change concerning American prisoner organ donation restrictions, a topic of increasing concern to him.

The Society had allotted forty-five minutes for his address, followed by fifteen minutes for questions. The text of his speech, with photos, would be released to the press right after his presentation, so there was sure to be intense interest from the media. His *NY Times* op-ed would appear the following morning; Zicheng wondered which media outlets would show the startling picture of his naked form following the hemicorporectomy.

Since their discussion and decision about their future, Lishan had been understanding, less tense, and helpful in the limited time she had available. They shared affection, but both knew the relationship would end soon.

As he drafted his speech, Zicheng and Lishan reviewed, revised, and re-reviewed the manuscript until they were satisfied. Zicheng then prepared his five-by-seven flashcards. His first practice run with the cards took nearly an hour. After two more rehearsals, he was down to forty minutes. Lishan said, "I want to help you with this presentation, but I hurt a little every time I realize that it may take us apart forever. Getting back to your presentation, I admire that you advocate for the use of organs from condemned people. I'm glad you're not putting in anything about my country's source of donors, the Uyghurs. I don't want you to bring shame to my country." Zicheng assured her that he would be sensitive, then emailed his manuscript to the Society.

Six weeks before going to New York, Zicheng met with Dr. Wong to resign his position as Assistant Surgeon. Zicheng's letter was effusive in his gratitude toward Wong and the Institute. Explaining his reasons, he wrote, "I have no complaints about you or the team or the Institute. Not only did you salvage my life, but you also gave me back my skills. The issue is cultural—I am an American first and foremost and cannot become Chinese in thinking, although I have tried. In America, I will tell the truth and the whole wonderful story. China and your Institute will get full credit for my rebirth and recovery. And thank you again. I hope you understand my reasons for leaving."

Wong read and then re-read the resignation letter. "I am disappointed by your decision to leave. If we increased your pay, would you consider staying?"

"No. The reason is not financial."

"I am sure you have thought this out thoroughly," said Wong. "I wish you every success. Do you have a new job arranged in the United States?"

"Not yet. I felt it was important to talk to you first. I'm not worried about finding a job. There are lots of vacancies." Dr. Wong looked solemn as they shook hands.

For the week before Zicheng's December departure, Dr. Li arranged a farewell banquet at Ku Lu Chi restaurant for Roger, Lishan, and the Institute senior staff. Doctors Wong and Li attended with their wives. At Zicheng's request, they invited the cottage cook, Fong. Dr. Wen flew in from Chengdu for the occasion. The banquet was sumptuous by Harbin standards— sweet and sour carp, cuttlefish roe soup, and braised intestines in brown sauce. Roger asked Lishan, "Why do they always think braised intestines are so special? They wouldn't appear on any Boston menu." His favorite items were the braised sea cucumber and braised prawns in oil. A small bottle of cognac stood in front of each plate, demonstrating that the Institute was honoring Zicheng. Dr. Wong proposed a toast to Zicheng and his new future in America; Zicheng responded with a salute to the team that had restored his life.

The next evening, when Lishan was at the hospital, Roger placed a call to his parents. "You know I'm coming back to the States for that talk in January. Well, guess what? I'm coming back to stay."

His father retrieved the phone Mildred had just dropped. "For real, son?"

Roger then explained his decision and promised to send his itinerary.

"There's a lot of joy today in Natick. Mom is dancing a little jig right now."

He arranged his travel as a one-way trip for Roger Scully. Lois Marshall arranged accommodation for three full days of media training before his address, scheduled for January 10. Accordingly, he set his itinerary to arrive in Denver on December 22 to get his skis and equipment from storage. He would fly to Boston on Christmas

Day to be with his parents. From December 28 through January 5, he would ski in Stowe, Vermont. Then he would have an overnight stop in Boston before his departure for Miami the next day.

Roger intended to meet up with a few close friends on the Christmas visit, and one of them promised to accompany him to Stowe. Swearing them to secrecy, he told them of the transplant and warned, "You'll be meeting a man who looks Chinese instead of a tall, handsome blond guy!" His friends expressed disbelief and could hardly contain their curiosity.

Explaining his itinerary to Lishan, he said, "Roger Scully is getting his life back."

Lishan frowned at him. "That hurts my feelings. You've had a life here in Harbin. You've had a life with me. It's as if you're dismissing so many months of your life. Dismissing me."

"I'm so sorry. I didn't mean it the way it sounded. It's just that I'm so relieved to be one person instead of two. It's hard to explain, and you've been so great through all this."

The *New York Times* was pressing to get an advance copy of his speech and his photograph. They felt that since they had agreed to run his op-ed the day after his talk, they deserved extra consideration in getting a prior view of his intended remarks. His agent obliged them with the op-ed text, and after a long discussion with Roger, a recent photo of him.

Zicheng's departure preparations were simple since his few personal possessions could travel as checked baggage and his new guitar as a carry-on. From his Harbin bank account, he transferred the equivalent of $10,000 to Lishan and sent the balance back to his Denver account.

When she learned of the monetary gift, Lishan protested, "That's not necessary. You don't owe me anything."

He shook his head to silence her protests. "It means you can keep the apartment through the end of the lease. And, of course, the furnishings and equipment are yours. The funds also help you move on to your next job, wherever that may be. Remember, we've promised to keep in touch. I'm interested in what happens in your life in the future. I'm sure you'll build more than chariots in your engineering career. Promise to stay in contact?"

"Of course. And you, too. Tell me you'll WeChat me, whatever you do in America," she said with tears.

"Of course, dear Lishan," Roger replied as they embraced. Roger noticed that Lishan's embrace was stiff and less than friendly.

On December 21, as Zicheng and Lishan were waiting in their apartment for the taxi to take him to the Harbin airport, their demeanors were strikingly different. Zicheng was full of nervous energy, pacing back and forth, going over his upcoming schedule, double-checking that he had packed everything he needed. Lishan sat in a chair, watching him fidget. "I'm sorry. But aren't you a little excited for me?" Zicheng asked.

"Yes, I *am* excited for you," she replied. "I just wish I could be excited for *us*. I'm going to miss you terribly."

Zicheng whirled toward her from the window, where he was keeping watch for the taxi. His lips quivered. "I have to go before I lose it. I owe you so much, and I still love you so much. Thank you for understanding."

They heard the taxi beep its horn. "Now go, *laowai*," Lishan whispered as she kissed him with tears streaming down her cheeks. He knew she was affectionately calling him a foreigner, which he would always be in China.

He was relieved when the plane set down in Hong Kong after the nine-hour flight. He barely noticed the dark-suited man board the plane before passengers began disembarking. As Roger approached the doorway, the man stood in front of him and asked, in English, "Your passport, please, Dr. Wu Zicheng." Assuming this was routine, Roger reached into his breast pocket and delivered the Chinese passport. The man nodded, turned away with the passport in hand, and left the aircraft ahead of a startled Roger, who followed.

"Hey, wait. What are you doing with my passport?"

"You just surrendered your Chinese passport. I assume Dr. Scully has another."

The man walked away quickly, accompanied by a uniformed and armed official. In a mild daze, Roger recovered his baggage and found his way to the airport hotel. He was relieved to have his U.S. passport returned by the Marriott check-in clerk. He could think of no one to call at this late hour. To vent his frustration, he sent an email to his attorney, Leung. After explaining the airport encounter, he finished with, "The bastards made sure they cut the cord this time. They won't see me again." He had a sleepless night, angry at the Chinese official.

Morning check-in with Delta was uneventful, as was U.S. immigration and boarding. The multi-stop trip was tiring, but as the plane finally landed at Denver International Airport, Roger felt the adrenaline overtake his tiredness. He rented a car, and on the way to his storage unit, he felt good at recognizing the streets near his apartment.

Seeing the familiar apartment building produced a wave of sadness. Roger recalled the day he and Joanne moved in, full of happiness and hope. Remembering the code to his storeroom, he retrieved his ski equipment. He looked around the compartment crowded with his Jeep and other belongings. There was nothing else he needed that day; the sight of the furniture brought him nearly to tears. He then returned to an airport hotel, where he collapsed. The next day was Christmas Eve Day, and he had made advance appointments to wrap up some minor business matters and then had free time to let his body adjust to the time difference.

However, that free time was interrupted by a WeChat call from Lishan, whose face revealed her agitation. "The Transplant Society released the program for the upcoming conference, and all hell has broken loose here," she reported. "The program identifies the keynote speaker as Wu Zicheng, and the place is crawling with reporters. That CNN guy is stalking me. Dr. Li called me to complain about how the media is hounding Dr. Wong. Everyone at the hospital is talking about us. A few people know your original identity, so I wouldn't be surprised if it gets leaked. I'm warning you, be prepared. I don't like living in this fishbowl."

Roger immediately recognized that the printed Transplant-Society program was misleading. Neither he nor Lois Marshall had told the conference organizers that he now wished to be known as Roger Scully; the program listed the speaker as Wu Zicheng. He did not worry about Harbin's concerns; he would tell his entire story at his talk on January 10. However, Roger knew his privacy was nearing its end.

"Lishan, be patient. All this will blow over in a few weeks, and besides, they're not interested in you, only me. Wong and Li have no reason to be upset. It's good advertising for the Institute." Lishan did not seem comforted by anything he said, and they ended their call with anxiety on both sides.

He had requested the Mountain of Snow Resort in Vermont to remove his name from the register; he was trying to keep a low profile. Roger hoped that his visit with his parents could go forward with no disruptions.

His parents were all smiles when they greeted him at Logan International. "This time, we recognized you," Mildred said, as she gave him a big hug and kiss, "but it's still going to take some time to get used to you in a different body. The nice thing is that we know we've got our son back as soon as you start talking. Merry Christmas, dear. I almost had a heart attack when you told us you were moving back to the States. It was one of the happiest days of my life."

"Merry Christmas to you both. It's great to be home," he replied.

"What I like is that you're once again Roger Scully," his dad chimed in, giving him a second hug. "I never did like that Zicheng moniker. What's your next step?"

"First, I'm going to take some time off and go skiing. At the Florida conference, I can start looking for a job. I haven't done anything about the job search yet, but I'm not worried. There's always a shortage of ER docs. They might even take me back in Denver."

"Are you still getting disability pay?"

"Oh, yes, but I'm sure it will stop the month after I speak in Florida. That's when I'll need a job."

"You should find a job in Boston. This is where you belong."

"We'll see where the job offers come from."

What a treat it was for Roger to see the Christmas tree in its usual spot, with its traditional ornaments. And when his mother brought out her homemade eggnog and special-recipe Irish Christmas Cake, the nostalgia started the tears rolling down his cheeks. That's all it took. As his dad handed him a handkerchief, Walter said, "I guess we might all have to use this," and the three gave way to tears of joy.

At dinner, his mother asked about Lishan. "Well, Mom, it's been painfully difficult for both of us, but we realized we needed to go in different directions for careers. Also, her family was a problem. They were not willing to accept a foreigner like me."

"Well, we would have accepted her here," said Walter, with a frown.

"Dad, it's different over there. Most Chinese are extremely xenophobic. And that, added to the career issues, finally led to our decision."

Mildred looked about to cry. "I hope you find another love real soon. Joanne was special; we loved her. And she would want you to be happy with another wife and start a family."

"Okay," Roger nodded, feeling tears well in his eyes, "let's just leave the topic if you don't mind."

Over the next few days, Roger shared his op-ed and conference speech with his parents, and they theorized how all their lives would change when he went public. "I don't relish the kind of media attention we're likely to get," his dad said.

His mom nodded in agreement. "You'll be a celebrity, but we don't want the limelight. I don't know how we're going to handle this."

Roger laughed, "Well, I'll bet your restaurant business picks up with all the people who hope to see the first brain transplant guy." But their concerns put an idea in his head. He telephoned Bill Wright to ask for recommendations for public relations people in Boston. Bill came up with two names, and Roger invited both to Natick to meet his parents. Roger explained that he would hire their favorite to be the family's official spokesperson so that all media requests would go through that individual. His parents were satisfied with all arrangements by the time he was ready for his ski trip.

His friend Ian picked him up for the trip to Stowe. After a handshake and a hug, Ian stood back, looked pensive, and stared at Roger's face. He moved around to get a profile view. "Great job on the plastic surgery. I worried you might look like someone out of Frankenstein."

Discussing their ski plans over dinner, Roger said, "Look, Ian, I think you should ski by yourself tomorrow. I have no idea how this new body will behave on the trails. There may not be any muscle memory at all. I'd better start on the bunny slope with some lessons before I get to the steeper stuff."

Roger was correct. Although he and the donor had almost identical height and body habitus, the boots and skis felt unfamiliar and clumsy. He arranged private lessons for the day, explaining to the instructor that he had not skied for many years, although his equipment was of recent vintage. After several falls and two near-collisions, he ended the day able to navigate the bunny slope safely. He retained the same instructor for more advanced lessons the following day.

Days two and three were a much better experience, as he mastered basic parallel turns and edge control. He could not explain to the instructor that he knew how to make the moves but had to think each one through instead of reflexively doing it. He graduated from the rope tow on the bunny hill to a Poma lift on a blue slope. He now felt competent to ski on his own, at least on easy runs.

Each night, he shared his dinner with Ian, a medical school classmate. After the third day of skiing, Roger was pleased to announce, "Good news. Today, Roger got most of his ski identity back!"

Ian smiled, raised a glass in a silent toast, and asked, "So, Roger, do you think of yourself as American or Chinese?"

"I tried being Chinese when I lived in Harbin. It didn't work. I was still being Roger and translating into Mandarin. I concluded I'd always feel like a foreigner and probably be treated as a foreigner by anyone who knew my story." Roger recounted, in considerable detail, his encounter with the police at the mosque. "I can't tell you how much more comfortable I am to be back in the U.S.A. as Roger Scully. No pretense, no acting."

His week at Stowe flew by. Roger felt the exhilaration of the movement, the wind on his face, the bright sun on the snow. After one fall, he learned to avoid even the small moguls. While on skis, he had no thought of Harbin, Bal Harbor, or his future. At night, with muscles aching from unaccustomed use, he fell asleep quickly.

On his final ski day, Roger realized he had not once called Lishan while in Vermont. Guilt nagged him. Without success, he tried to reach her that evening and the next morning. But at the same time, he wondered how Lishan would fit into his everyday life in America. In Harbin, they had created a narrowly focused living, built on their connections with the Institute. Hard work and long hours had almost made any social life impossible. He had ignored her disapproval of "stupid American politics" while she never answered his questions about the Chinese repression of Uyghurs. Their cultural differences didn't matter much in that context. But living in America would magnify their differences.

His mind was distracted by two attractive emails. Lois suggested he accept an offer for a *60 Minutes* interview the day after the Miami address. A message from Human Resources at the University Hospital in Denver said they would like one of their representatives, a Dr. Smith, to meet with him in Miami during the conference. He agreed, thinking it would be about returning to his old job. With some excitement, but without success, he tried to call Lishan. She had not returned his three previous voice mails. His guilt was fading like his mild sunburn.

Roger left Stowe with satisfaction at the experience. He stopped overnight in Natick to deposit his ski equipment and dined on lobster with his parents at the local Legal Seafood. Lois Marshall met him at the Miami airport, then drove him to a Marriott in Miami, next to the media center for his training, well away from the convention site at Bal Harbor. She had preregistered him at the hotel and arranged with the manager to conceal his presence. That night, Roger enjoyed a room service hamburger and fries while he watched a hockey game on TV.

The next three days proved intriguing. Roger had not understood the strategies involved in doing a press interview and various skills for television. The training in the television studio also allowed him to rehearse his address to the conference. He had qualms about the reaction to his talk but felt confident in his ability to deliver the speech.

Roger got up at 6 a.m. to call Lishan on WeChat before his big day. She was tired from her long day and showed little interest in his recount of the media training. She asked, "Does that mean you're going to be a TV person and not a doctor?" He reassured her and suggested she watch CNN for coverage of his speech.

CHAPTER 17

Promptly at 8:30 a.m., Lois Marshall appeared at his suite for the move to Bal Harbor. "You're in the auditorium from 9 until 10. I arranged a room for a press conference from 10 until 11."

"I'm nervous about my address. The program lists me as Wu Zicheng, MD. No one there is expecting Roger Scully. They all think Wu Zicheng has always been Chinese."

"So you'll give them a nice surprise. Your media preparation went well. You can be confident about your presentation. The meeting with the press is important. Otherwise, reporters will harass you all day."

"How many will there be?"

"Hard to say. Probably a dozen; there might be twenty. Right up-front, I'll identify any topic we consider off-limits. That'll make it easier for you and will give *60 Minutes* some new things to talk about."

"Then what? Do I get a break?" Roger asked.

"I'll give you an hour off, and then we'll get lunch somewhere private. After that, you're meeting with two publishing houses that are pitching you to write a book. You can be a sole author, ghostwriter, or cowriter."

"You didn't mention a book deal."

Lois replied, "Sorry, but think about it. The publisher can find an appropriate writer to work with you if you want to go that route. There's a lot of money in a book deal."

"If I don't find a job quickly, I may need the book deal. Is that it for the day? I had an email from the University of Colorado asking me to have dinner with Doctor Ruben Smith. I don't recognize the name, but I presume it's about a job."

"That sounds important, so I'll try to reschedule George Maclin."

"George who?"

"Maclin, he represents the best speaker's bureau in the business."

Roger shook his head. "I never imagined myself as a celebrity, but media training made me understand the importance of a press conference. I hadn't thought of a speaker's bureau. Why that?"

"You must understand that, like it or not, you *are* a celebrity," Lois replied. "I'm here to help manage that. The speaker's bureau will let you pick and choose your speaking engagements and negotiate your fees, which could be substantial."

"But what would I speak about? I can't keep giving the same speech as I do here," he said.

"Most invitations will be from those who want details about your transplant. However, you also have a cause: you're trying to get organs to sick people from donors who want to donate while in prison or condemned to death. You have a chance to do well by doing good. So remember both topics when you do the *60 Minutes* interview in CBS's Miami studio. In the afternoon, I've invited representatives of the-transplant organizations to meet you. They have been calling me because they see your advocacy as important to their needs."

"I think brain surgery is easier," Roger sighed. "Let's discuss the press conference limitations: no family background or childhood stuff. Let's keep to the facts of the accident, the surgeries, my recovery, and the job I just left. I'll tell them I've now moved back to the States. Someone might pick up on that and offer me a job."

"What about capital punishment questions?"

"I'm against it, but I'm prepared to say my donor was a condemned-to-death prisoner."

Lois agreed to the limitations, and they left for the conference at the Hyatt Regency in Bal Harbor. Before their taxi had stopped, they saw the protestors. Ten men and women were picketing the hotel with signs such as, "Stop killing people for their organs" and "Kill capital punishment." Two opposing demonstrators held signs, "Complete your organ donor card." Four television cameramen waited on the sidewalk. Lois instructed the driver to divert to the hotel's rear service entrance to avoid the scene.

Inside the hotel, several uniformed security personnel stood throughout the corridors and outside the conference room. Ten men and women wearing PRESS badges sat among the auditorium crowd; white men over age forty filled most seats. Roger strode to the stage steps and spotted the apparent chairman, Wilbur Ross, who was looking about for his speaker. When Roger appeared, the chair gave a relieved smile. "Thank you so much for coming, Dr. Wu. Most of us in the transplant community never thought this surgery would happen, but it's here. And we have the added advantage that a surgeon was the recipient. We can't wait to hear the details."

"I should have told you earlier, but please introduce me as Roger Scully because I'm now using my previous identity."

Ross looked startled but gave a shrug and confirmed Roger's biographical details as they waited for the audience to settle.

The chairman's introduction of Roger was unusual. "We are honored today to have as our guest speaker, not Doctor Wu Zicheng, but Dr. Roger Scully, an American MD, board-certified in emergency medicine, licensed in Colorado, and finally, the first recipient of a corporeal transplant." Heads leaned forward, murmurs erupted, and Roger noticed that hardly anyone in the audience was looking at the chairman—they were staring at him. After thanking the chairman, Roger projected a previous photo of himself labeled, "Roger Scully, MD, Director of Emergency Services, University of Colorado Hospital." The picture was dated two years earlier and bore no resemblance to the speaker. Without commenting on the slide, Roger started, "I stand before you at the apex of the transplant movement that began over 100 years ago with the first corneal transplants. We owe much to pioneers Medowar and Starzl. They made possible today's complex organ transplants, such as faces and hands."

Turning to his personal history, he recounted his crush injury in Tibet, the attempts to salvage at least stumps for legs, and then the hemicorporectomy. At that point, he projected the slide (from Lishan's phone), showing his naked body. The audience gasped and started to murmur. Roger left the image on the screen. "You have now seen two pictures of the former Roger Scully. It's not often your guest speaker shows a nude photo of himself." He laughed, and the audience responded with smiles and nods.

He continued, "Some months before my injury, Dr. Dengwei Wong of Harbin University Medical School published an account of an operation in which he kept a transplanted head alive for several days. That operation took eighteen hours. Most of you are aware of that report and the consternation it caused. The criticism did not deter Dr. Wong, who has since continued to perfect his team's techniques, which have made possible a corporeal transplant, of which I am an example. I use that term rather than brain transplant because the brain owner is the recipient. The body is the donor organism." He went on to describe in detail the pre-operative preparations of donor and patient, the surgery (including micro-robotics), and the postoperative care. He gave full credit to the foresight, skill, and tenacity of Dr. Wong and his team.

"At the end of my transplant, another surgical team salvaged both corneas, both kidneys, lungs, liver, and heart to benefit seven additional patients from my former body. They didn't waste a thing!

"They've gone on to do several more corporeal transplants and have an 80 percent success rate. At present, they're limited only by the surgeons' available time. From all over the world, including the United States, patients are applying for transplants." The audience stirred with many muffled discussions.

"I faced a difficult decision. Should I have a life like this?" (he pointed to the Chengdu slide) "or take a chance with Dr. Wong?" He showed another picture of himself, this time in the chariot. "Here, you see what we called my chariot. I could move around, but I admit that I wanted as much of my old life back as modern medicine could provide.

"I think most of you would have made the same choice as I did. I have never regretted my decision.

"So where do they get the donors? Most of you know that China has a vigorous transplant program, in part because of the ready availability of organs from condemned prisoners. Their high rate of capital punishment produces thousands of potential donors. Persons condemned to death have a choice: donate their organs and die under an anesthetic or be shot in the head. Families must also consent to any organ donation, so the Chinese argue they obtain informed consent.

"For tomorrow's *New York Times,* I wrote an op-ed piece giving my views on a transplant from prisoner donors. Although I absolutely oppose capital punishment, I vigorously advocate availability of all organs from individuals condemned to capital punishment. Corporeal transplants will be rare, but one donated body could save several lives. Remember—we're talking about body donors who would have given consent to this process. I understand your anguish when a sick person dies under your care while waiting for an organ. No state or federal law prohibits the use of prisoner organs, but state and federal administrations won't allow it. There is also a reason to allow prisoners to donate organs without undergoing capital punishment. Healthy donors can give a kidney or a lobe of the liver. Prisoners who would make such a donation should receive compensation—money or time off their sentence.

"As an association, I hope you will continue to pressure state and federal lawmakers to enact legislation promoting prisoner organ donations. Thank you for the opportunity to share my experiences and views. I admire the work you do and hope that changed regulations will ensure greater success in that work in the future." He put up a slide showing his email address.

The audience stood and applauded loudly. The chairman then invited two noted medical ethicists to each deliver a five-minute presentation. The first criticized the idea of prisoner organ donation, fearing that it would strengthen the argument for capital punishment. The second ethicist agreed with Dr. Scully on the humanitarian grounds of doing the most good for the most people.

After the allotted fifteen minutes for questions, the chairman had trouble stopping the spirited clamor from the audience. Roger had struck a nerve. Lois and security personnel escorted him through a crowded aisle to an exit.

About thirty reporters and camera crews crowded the press room following his speech. Surgeons who had attended the conference tried to cram into the press briefing, but security kept them out while Lois tried to keep order. All of the questioners had listened to his address that morning. A few questions related to the surgical procedure, but there was more interest in personal issues. Reporters asked:

"What's it like to wake up in another man's body?"

"It takes a bit of getting used to. The first week was the most difficult."

"Have you encountered any discrimination against Asians?"

"None I've been aware of."

"Do you have any regrets about your decision?"

"None whatsoever. The operation freed me from a useless body with no career prospects and limited mobility."

"Do you feel out of place now in the U.S.?"

"To the contrary, I feel I am home at last."

"Are you going to move back to the States?"

"I have moved back. I'm here to stay."

Roger was relieved that he and Lois had predicted virtually all the questions. His back stiffened at questions regarding Chinese prisoners. He refused to defend the Chinese use of capital punishment.

"Are you grateful to the donor?"

"Of course, yes."

"Do you realize that California has more than 700 persons on death row?"

"Yes, I know the statistics."

"Won't advocates of the death penalty use your suggestions about organ donation to justify more convictions?"

"I hope not, but I have no control over future judges and juries. I think the ethicists discussed the opposing viewpoints this morning."

"Is it true that Wong in Harbin is now offering corporeal transplants to ALS patients?"

"Not specifically targeting that population, but they are doing some ALS patients at present."

"What is Harbin charging for a corporeal transplant?"

"I have no knowledge of the finances and no clue about payment."

"You are a widower. Are you going to get married again?"

"Those kinds of questions are off-limits."

To Roger's relief, Lois ended the session and thanked the press for coming. Over lunch with Roger, she expressed her pleasure at how he had handled himself in every instance. She confirmed a breakfast meeting tomorrow with George Maclin of the speaker's bureau. "So, what's going on with your dinner tonight?"

"I'm a little shocked. After Ruben Smith emailed me to confirm our dinner, I looked him up. He's the new president of the University of Colorado. He was in the audience today."

"Sounds exciting, so you need some rest. I'll call you just before 3 o'clock when the first publisher arrives."

In his suite, he kicked off his shoes and stretched out on the bed. He regretted his appointments with the publishers. *Too many meetings today.* He was confused about the upcoming meeting with the president of the University of Colorado. Roger had neither time nor energy to worry about it. He immediately fell asleep.

An hour later, Lois Marshall called him. "I know it's early for the publishers' meeting, but I just had a call from CNN. They want to interview you and then retain you as a special consultant. They don't pay for the interview, but the consultant gig would be a retainer, and they would call you when a relevant news story breaks. For those episodes, you would get a fee each time you appear. Can I get your authority to negotiate with them?"

"I suppose it doesn't hurt to talk. I never thought of anything like that. Listen to them, but don't make any deals. I'm trying to sort out my future job and career, so I'll take it slow in making any commitments. Do I still have the *60 Minutes* interview tomorrow?"

"Yes, they're doing a segment on transplant programs in the U.S. and want to hear your views on organ availability. I don't know if you are aware that there is a bit of a scandal at the moment concerning the inefficiency of the not-for-profit companies that have sprung up to try to promote organ donations and facilitate organ distribution. Events like Steve Job's liver transplant angered families of patients who have waited much longer."

"I'm glad you arranged the media training program. It looks like I'll need it. See you in twenty minutes?"

"Yes, same room as the press conference. I booked it for the day. See you there."

Lois had arranged for both publishers to have twenty minutes each with her and Roger. The two tossed a coin for the first appointment.

Theresa Myer won the toss. "Dr. Scully, I'll be quick. You have a story that will make an inspiring book. I watched your BBC interview. I managed to get into the conference. Ordinarily, someone writes a book, then finds an agent, and the agent brings it to us. I'm suggesting we short-circuit that process. I can recommend a talented writer who will listen to your story and get it down with accuracy and sensitivity. You'll control the book and be the author. How does that sound?"

"Is that what you call a ghostwriter?"

"That term is used, but let's make no mistake. It's your story. It's your book."

"And how do I make money on this?"

"Well, if you agree to the situation, there's a variety of ways. Assume you go ahead with my suggestion. We introduce you to the writer, and you make a contract with them. Typically, you'll pay them 20 to 30 percent of your earnings from the book, including the advance. Because you don't have an agent, you save the 15 percent commission they usually take. It's a good deal because the writer does all the work, and you stand to make a lot of money. There might also be TV or movie deals after the book that will add to your take."

"What time frame are we talking about?"

"Well, because the story is fresh, I suggest you move on it quickly. A good writer like the one I would recommend will get the book's first draft in four to six months. That would trigger payment of your advance. One of our editors would work with you and your writer to finish the book over three or four months. Figure a year from now to have the book hit the shelves."

"How much money are we talking about?"

"I'm not authorized to give you a guarantee at this time, but you could easily clear half to a million dollars or more."

"That's serious change, but I have to think about this. You'll have to give me time to sort out my life before we start writing about it."

Lois Marshall spoke up. "I think Dr. Scully has the information he needs for the moment. I have your card. I'll get back to you when we have made any decisions, one way or another. And you will contact me and not bother the good doctor, okay?"

"That's great. Dr. Scully, you have an inspiring story. I wish you well in your new life."

For the second publisher, Roger had little enthusiasm or interest. Until he had settled on a job, he would not make any commitment concerning a book. That interview was a repeat of the first, with minor differences. Lois and Roger listened politely. Lois asked a few questions and closed out the meeting. Roger saw little to differentiate one over the other.

CHAPTER 18

After Roger met Dr. Smith outside the dining room, the hostess led them to a corner table. Over drinks and after complimentary comments on Roger's conference presentation, Smith got down to business.

"As you know, I'm the new president of the University of Colorado at Denver. You're probably wondering why I asked for this meeting."

"Well, yes," Roger nodded.

"A university president has two major functions. One is to raise money, and the other is to recruit faculty. I'm not here to raise money. I'm here to ask you to come back to Denver. We're starting the Life Prolongation Institute, and we need a director. We call it the LPI for short. That Institute will run a major transplant research and treatment program. Not just organ transplants; we also want to develop artificial organs. So, there'll be implants and research to develop new technologies."

Roger's ears perked up at the mention of an institution that would do both research and transplants, plus develop artificial organs. What a combination! He wanted to learn more and what his role might be.

"Sounds interesting, but why me?"

"Transplant surgeons are hard to find and even tougher to hire. Right after I heard your presentation today, I called a few members of our search committee. When I told them about you that confirmed what we knew about you, they asked me to talk to you about heading up our new Institute."

Roger was startled. "Well, I'm flattered, but I'm not the world's most noted transplant surgeon. I've done that surgery just for the past year."

Smith smiled. "You're a known commodity in Denver. You were not doing research, but you ran an outstanding emergency department. You have good people skills and were highly respected. The residents who rotated through your department were uniformly positive in their reviews. You're a very high-energy person. Now you've had experience at the Harbin Institute, which leads the world in transplant research. We want to challenge their leadership and excel in both clinical and technological research."

Smith continued, "We already have good neuroscience and immunology programs, and the engineering faculty is strong in biomedical. The director will be a tenured professor responsible for building a teaching and research program. Your first task would be to find and hire qualified faculty."

"The job sounds like a big challenge," Roger responded. "Working at Harbin has given me an interest in doing research. But I also like to treat patients. I have several questions. First, would I have an opportunity to do surgery?"

"I don't see why not. That is something you would negotiate with the surgical departments and hospitals."

"Is this a basic science or clinical science position?" Roger asked.

"Interesting question. For some reason, that hasn't come up before. What's your thought?"

Roger replied, "As a clinician, I lean toward making it a clinical department, but it could go either way. I'd feel more comfortable with clinical."

"Then let's assume that is where we'll put it."

"Can we do animal research in the new institute?" Roger asked.

"Animal research? Provided you treat animals humanely, and the research passes our Animal Health Committee, there are no restrictions."

"Could the Institute afford to buy state-of-the-art robotic equipment?"

"You asked about equipment that I assume is expensive. The group funding the Institute has made it clear that they intend to provide large equipment grants to ensure we're competitive with the rest of the world. Until we have a leader, we can't estimate the equipment or money we will need."

"Who pays for all this?" Roger asked.

Smith smiled again. "Good question. Colorado led the country in medical marijuana legislation. No pun intended, but it's a growth industry; their CEOs want to funnel some profits into medical research. After a lot of discussions, they came up with the idea of the Life Prolongation Institute."

"Fascinating," said Roger. After another hour of discussion, Roger had heard enough to pique his interest. "I'll come to Colorado to take a look. How can we arrange that?"

"This being a university, naturally we have a search committee, so I can't offer you a job just yet. I know they want to talk with you. I'd like you to make the trip as soon as possible."

The two men quickly agreed on a visit ten days later, which allowed Smith time to arrange the interview appointments. Roger had never met a search committee, so this was a new challenge. He was giddy with excitement. He was happy that he would have time to do a little skiing before the meeting.

That evening, he called his parents and told them about the probable offer. They sounded ecstatic; Roger warned them that the deal was not sealed and had to be kept confidential. He asked them to ship his skis to Denver.

He stayed for the final days of the conference. He was becoming more abreast of the very fast-moving transplant field. He met and had drinks with several surgeons he now viewed as colleagues. It felt good to be back in the States and among a group that treated him as one of their peers.

Over breakfast, Roger met Maclin of the speaker's bureau and listened to the pitch, "Right now, I'm negotiating for a job as a professor. I can't tell you where, but I might not have time for speaking gigs around the country. "

"Good luck with the negotiations. The title of professor will increase your value as a speaker. It's also good publicity for your new department when you're looking to recruit faculty."

Roger agreed to call Maclin when he had an academic appointment.

Lois had arranged for him to meet leaders of several organizations promoting and recruiting donors for transplant programs. The ALS Association also attended. "Go for it, Doctor Scully; you can help us a lot," was a common comment. Every organization voiced its support for his plea to allow prisoners to volunteer, and they all committed to political action at the state and national levels.

For the rest of the day, Roger attended demonstrations and workshops concerning new surgical techniques or anti-rejection drugs. No one discussed long-term survival. Surgeons reported results only in terms of thirty or ninety-day survival when they evaluated a new operation. He resolved that an early hire might be a statistician or epidemiologist if he landed the Denver job. None were present here, but someone should evaluate the long-term survival and effects. While listening to presentations, he was mentally scouting for potential faculty members. Professional conferences are prime hunting grounds.

Roger arranged a flight to Denver six days before his appointment with the search committee so that he would have a chance to ski. He gloried in the week at Snowmass, though the famous knee-deep powder severely challenged his still-developing skills. He enjoyed the après-ski socializing and tried flirting outrageously with several women. When two consecutive women rebuffed him immediately, he wondered if his Asian appearance was to blame. He had almost forgotten Lishan.

On Sunday, he drove to Denver to check in at the familiar Brown Palace Hotel, with its eight-story atrium lobby. Dining alone on rack of venison, he treated himself to a pre-dinner Manhattan and two glasses of a fine Pinot Noir to steel himself for the appointments tomorrow.

Back in his room, he had difficulty concentrating on the hockey game. *What will they ask me tomorrow? What are they looking for?* Sleep did not come easily that night.

Monday morning, he first met the dean. Following that appointment, he saw two associate deans and the director of the neuroscience program. After lunch, when he met with the professor of biomedical engineering, his brain lit up. The man lamented his difficulty in finding engineers with medical degrees. That statement brought memories of Lishan back into his thoughts.

His final appointment of the afternoon was with Bill Reiker, the professor and chair of the Department of Surgery. Reiker was about sixty, wearing a stiff white coat over a starched white shirt and conservative tie. After a handshake, he got right to the point. "I'm a bit puzzled. Is your transplant department going to do surgery?"

Showing his surprise, Roger answered, "Well, not as a department, but I anticipate that I and others I appoint will work with the appropriate surgical departments. As an extreme example, if there ever is a brain transplant, I would work with the neurosurgeons and vascular guys."

"Looking at your CV, I see two years of general surgery residency before you switched to Emergency Medicine. Do I have that right?"

"You're correct. My interests changed," Roger said.

"But no neurosurgery rotation, I assume, but you would work on a brain transplant?"

Roger felt defensive. "But I'm the only one here who has scrubbed on brain transplants and am familiar with the technique. I can teach the neurosurgeons a few things."

"Right. I see that. But would the neurosurgeons admit the patient, or are you looking for admission privileges yourself?" asked Reiker.

"I haven't thought of that issue, but I assume the patient would be on the neurosurgical service," Roger answered. "I would hope to have admitting privileges as courtesy staff."

"I may be sounding bureaucratic, but the issue is important. Our teaching hospitals are divided by specialties, and I can't quite envision a transplant department having its own space. You're going to be recruiting faculty. What kind of people are you seeking?"

Roger brightened. "I'm already looking at some candidates working on brain science. One is growing brainoids that have a potential for transplant. The other has already published in the field of NITs, the neurologic-information technologies. We need to take their laboratory and animal work to the patients. We have to find more sources to replace organs. We may have to grow new organs, manufacture electronic or mechanical substitutes, and change how we organize our tissue donors."

Reiker smiled, "I remember when I was Senior Resident, and Starzl did the first kidney and liver transplant. We could see a new day in surgery. I'm not criticizing you or your institute. I question where you are putting it and what your personal role is going to be. That said, good luck with it."

He stood up to indicate the interview was ended. Roger took the outstretched hand, said a brief thank you, and left for his next appointment at the Emergency Room. On his long walk through the halls, he pondered the Reiker interview. While it was not entirely positive, the surgeon had raised some pertinent points. *I wonder if my shop should be in the Basic Sciences Division? Should I try for a cross-appointment in Neurosurgery?*

The ER visit was a pleasant change. The current director, George Hill, was someone he had trained and mentored. Roger said, "I'm here looking at a job to head a new Institute. If I get the job, can you get me an appointment to your ER so I can do the occasional shift to keep my skills?"

Hill smiled, "You're still listed in our department. We never took your name off the roster. Can I use you this weekend?" He accompanied the question with a laugh to indicate he was not serious.

"Maybe not this weekend. I don't have the job yet, but I'll be glad to do one or two shifts a month if I'm here."

One of the veteran nurses greeted him with a hug, albeit after a long stare at him and the question, "Dr. Scully?" All staff smiled with pleasure that one of their own was moving up.

He toured the entire medical campus. He was aware that the three-day visit had a dual purpose: to impress him enough to make him want the job and to vet him for the position. The visit had achieved its first goal. Roger was impressed by the knowledge and enthusiasm shown by the professionals he had met. Here was a perfect opportunity to do both research and patient treatment. He would also have a platform from which to influence the development of innovative transplant technologies. He was not yet convinced the committee would offer him the job; Reiker's interview left him concerned.

The interview process culminated on Wednesday morning. For almost two hours, the search committee grilled him about his impressions of the visit, his vision for the future of the new Institute, and any concerns he might have. He seemed to excite the group by suggesting that future transplants would almost certainly include organoids, specifically brain tissue grown in the laboratory. Scientists had already succeeded with cultures that developed brain-like structures with connecting neurons. Roger explained that such "mini-brains" could replace brain tissue destroyed by tumor, trauma, or surgery. From the surprised look and a single question, he deduced that these men had never heard of brainoids. Their frowns and concerned looks made him wonder about being too radical in his proposals. Undeterred, Roger discussed innovations in neural information technologies (NITS) and advanced prostheses. The group looked startled when he mentioned his own implanted neural sensors. He hoped his remarks demonstrated that he was the visionary the committee was seeking, although the committee's faces showed no emotion that he could discern.

Dr. Reiker raised the only threatening question. "Yesterday, I raised my concern over your clinical activity. Have you given any more thought to that?"

"Yes. Thank you for asking. You suggested my Institute would be better placed with the Basic Sciences. I'm not against that, but I will be more comfortable with the clinicians. I'm a practicing doctor more than a scientist. I don't want a separate clinical department for transplants. Perhaps an appropriate mix of cross-appointments will solve the issue."

The committee had no more questions. The Dean asked, "Dr. Scully, do you have any other questions for the group?" Seeing Roger shake his head, he continued, "Then, if you don't mind, perhaps you can wait in my lobby outside the room. You'll find coffee and sodas there; we won't be long."

The twenty-minute wait seemed like an hour, and Roger paced the lobby. He realized his heart was beating fast, and he unconsciously crossed his fingers, then laughed at himself for doing so. He played with his cell phone, aware that a jury inside was deciding his life. Would Reiker vote against his appointment?

Suddenly, individuals filed out, with parting comments such as, "Thank you for coming," or "it was a pleasure to meet you." He could not read them. The Dean, the last person to exit, invited him into his private office.

"Well, Dr. Scully, will you take the job?" the Dean asked.

"Are you offering it to me?"

"Yes, I am. The committee was unanimous, and everyone hopes you will join the faculty."

"And the salary?" he asked, buoyed by the offer.

The Dean named an amount almost double what Roger had been getting as director of the hospital emergency room.

"That's acceptable to me, thank you," said Roger, as they shook hands. "Am I still in the Clinical Science division, or do I get moved?"

The Dean nodded, "Why don't we meet with the Vice President of Health Sciences and the Associate Deans, Clinical and Basic Science. Among us, I'm sure we can sort it out. My office will arrange the meeting. Let's not hold up your appointment over that."

"When does the job start?"

"The position is open now, but you have a big transition to make. What about a March 1st starting date?" said a smiling Dean.

"I can make that work," Roger replied.

Once back in his hotel room, Roger e-mailed his parents, confirming his new appointment. He texted Lishan, "Urgent matter. Please call me ASAP." He assumed she would see the text when she arose at 6 a.m. He then texted Will Willoughby, his best friend in Denver.

"In town. Take you and Susanne for dinner tonight?"

Within minutes his phone rang. "Roger, what are you doing? Why didn't you warn us you were coming to town? Of course, we'll have dinner with you. What's happening? We heard about your Miami talk, but you haven't been answering any of my e-mails before or since."

"I'm sorry and embarrassed. You're one of several people I need to get back to. I'll explain it all tonight, and dinner will be on me to make amends."

"No need for that, but we'll be glad to see you."

"I'm moving back to Denver. I'll tell you more about it over dinner. How about 7 tonight at the Brown Palace?"

"Fantastic news. Susanne and I look forward to seeing you."

At almost precisely 6 p.m., Lishan called. "Zicheng, is there a problem?"

"Something exciting, Lishan. I got the job I told you about as the director of the new Institute. But get this, there is a Department of Biomedical Engineering. I spent an hour with the department chair, and he is desperately looking for engineers with medical degrees. You're the ideal candidate. Would you consider it?"

"Wow, you do surprise me. I just woke up. Congratulations on the new position. I know you were excited about it. I have an appointment for an interview in Xinhua in two weeks to see about a job when the residency is over in June. If I moved to Denver, would I be working for you?"

"Not at all. The Department of Biomedical Engineering is in the Engineering Faculty. My Institute is in the Faculty of Medicine. Do you mind if I give Hal Osler your name and e-mail? He's the chair I was talking about."

"He can contact me. I have some reservations about looking at a job in the USA, but you know about that," Lishan replied.

"Give it some serious thought, Lishan. Have you time to talk now?"

"No, I have a scrub in twenty minutes with no time for breakfast. Let's talk later. I'll text my schedule to you. And Zicheng, I still love you." Before he could reply, Lishan had hung up.

Roger entertained the Willoughbys through dinner with the story of his journey from hemicorporectomy to being a successful surgeon. Wide-eyed, Will said, "Gee, you should write a book about your life and how it feels to be one person made up of two individuals."

"Great idea. I could call it *Chimera* because that's what I am."

"Call it what? Wasn't that some mythical Greek thing?"

"Yes, but the biologists have taken the term, and it now means an organism with more than one kind of DNA. That's me."

When Roger returned to his room at 9 p.m., he had exhausted the adrenaline supply that had fueled him all day. Lishan had texted to suggest a call at 8 a.m. Denver time. He texted his agreement and fell into bed without brushing his teeth.

Eight hours of sleep and a shower gave Roger a new life. When he called Lishan at 8 o'clock, he had finished breakfast and was enjoying a second cup of coffee.

"First, tell me about your new job."

With much enthusiasm, he explained the Institute, its funding, and the freedom he anticipated. He was particularly enthusiastic about his meeting with Hal Osler. "He and I ran out of time talking. You know, I think the future of transplants will also involve artificial organs. Look at the neural net of sensors I have inside my skull. I hope you'll talk to him."

"All right. Give him my contact information. Zicheng, don't get your hopes up too high. You know I have a real problem when I think about going to America." They signed off in a friendly fashion. Roger was encouraged that she might consider Denver.

He went off to his morning appointment with Jan Steiner, the Associate Dean of Administration. They spent almost an hour reviewing space, budget, hiring policies, and medical school politics. He would officially start in three weeks. A new life awaited.

CHAPTER 19

March 1. With some trepidation and slight nausea, Roger Scully walked from the parking structure to his new office. The previous week, the University had issued his picture and press release concerning the appointment. The public now knew he was the recipient of a donor body. The cold March wind burned his cheeks as he anticipated his first day as professor and chair, Department of Transplant Surgery and Director, Life Prolongation Institute at the University of Colorado. He had been in teaching hospitals for virtually all his medical career, but he never imagined that he would be a full professor at one.

Doctor Scully had immediately impacted the transplant world by articulating some of the problems and prospects for more transplant surgery. In China, he had pioneered corporeal transplant for victims of ALS, a uniformly fatal disease. Here in the U.S., Roger had renewed the public debate about condemned prisoners having the right to donate their organs while in prison or at the time of execution. In this, he had emphasized the need for dying patients to get transplants and the challenge of cardiothoracic surgeons pleading for more organs. He was now in a position where he had a voice, an organization, and probably the budget to make a difference.

He had moved from obscurity as a transplant surgeon in Harbin, China, to lead an institute at a prestigious American medical school. Two weeks earlier, he had visited Denver to examine his new office and work with the University administration to hire an administrative assistant and complete the bureaucratic paperwork concerning his employment. He was preoccupied with a question. *Am I up to the job?*

As he rounded the corner to the quad in front of his office, he saw them. There, in front of Roger's building, a group of ten students picketed with placards. Two of the signs were in Mandarin characters, presumably for any Chinese or Hong Kong media that might pick up the story. The remainder read things such as, "Uyghur Lives Matter, Stop Chinese Organ Farming, and Don't Reward Racial Injustice."

A startled Roger turned up his coat collar, increased his pace, and strode by the group while avoiding eye contact. He was almost at the stairs.

"Look, there's the bastard!" A clamor arose from the group as he reached the stairs. He was up and then into the building before anyone could intercept him. In the lobby, he noted the building directory now included his name and position. A uniformed security guard watched the demonstrators outside. Roger eschewed the elevator and sprinted up the staircase to the second floor. At the end of the hall, there was a glass door with the black letters Department of Transplant Surgery. He had arrived. He found his office entrance locked, and as he fumbled with the unfamiliar key, Marsha opened the door from inside.

"Hi, Marsha," he said with a sigh of relief.

"Good morning, boss. Welcome to the University and the home of free speech. They were assembling when I arrived, but I didn't have time to warn you. I'm keeping the door locked."

"What happens now?"

"It's a little early for the Dean or Vice President to show up, but I imagine you'll hear soon. Would you like coffee?" she asked, leading him into the small kitchen. Roger was pleasantly surprised to note the Peet's coffee beans, a grinder, and the French press he had requested.

"Good idea. This scene is not how I imagined my first day."

Marsha, his new administrative assistant, had started the week before to organize the office with supplies, computers, etc. She had previously worked in the Department of Pediatrics, so she was familiar with University procedures and protocols. She was ready with a list of questions for him to decide, starting with the stationery and business card layout, conference room furniture, and his preferences concerning telephone call screening.

As Marsha made her coffee after him, he asked, "How much do you know about me?"

She replied, "Not all that much. I've seen the press release the administration put out. Your photo made you look handsome. Everyone is curious to see the white man in the Chinese body. I didn't put that very well, but there is a lot of curiosity. Oh, and by the way, you need to prepare a CV for the file. I'll get a lot of requests for it, and the Dean's office didn't send one over."

"Let's sit down with our coffee, and I'll give you my background. None of it is secret." With that, he went through his life history, including the New England childhood, his medical school and residency training, his previous Denver ER work, and then his accident in Tibet. He briefly summarized his corporeal transplant; the news media had preceded him on that story.

As he was ending his story, Marsha answered the phone. "Yes, he's here," and handed it to him, explaining, "Dr. Hamilton, Vice

President of Health Sciences." He switched to speakerphone, so Marsha could hear.

"Good morning, Professor Scully. I'm afraid your welcome today was unexpected. Let me explain. On Friday, a Professor Shan sent me an email protesting your appointment on the grounds of Chinese repressions of Uyghurs. I called him, and we agreed to meet with you this week to discuss the matter. Today I called him as soon as I heard about the protestors, but he's not in yet and not expected until after 10. Typical liberal arts academic. So we'll wait until I hear."

"Who's Shan?" asked Roger.

"Sociologist. Made tenure last year. Reputation as left-wing, but with solid publication record. Don't do anything until you hear from me. Stay out of sight of the protestors."

"I'll be careful. I won't leave my office until I hear from you." As he ended the call, he threw up his hands in disbelief.

He opened his computer calendar and was surprised to see more than a dozen appointments for the current week.

Marsha explained, "I took the liberty of making these appointments for people who called. I can change any of them if they interfere with other plans of which I'm unaware. I prioritized them. In an hour, first on the list is Doctor Jan Schneider, Associate Dean for Administration here in the medical school. You met him a few weeks ago when he suggested you hire me. He can be useful because he controls the money. He also knows more about the politics of this place than anyone else." She continued to review his appointment with a series of senior academics, many of whom he had met on the Search Committee. "Tomorrow morning, you see the Dean, and an hour after, you're to meet Doctor Hamilton, the Vice President of Health Sciences that you just talked with. You'll notice a Friday afternoon meeting for clinical department heads. That meeting is on the first Friday of every month; all department heads are expected to be there. It usually goes from 2 until 4."

Roger was surprised at the levels of administration. He had never considered such a bureaucracy in a medical school.

Together they created what Roger considered an embarrassingly short CV. He was sure his resume would be the least impressive of all the clinical professors. As they finished, Dr. Hamilton called back.

Dr. Hamilton did not waste time with pleasantries. "We have an awkward problem, Professor Scully. Today from the Sociology Department, Professor Shan wrote a letter to the University President, complaining that hiring you supports Chinese policies on capital punishment, Uyghur repression, and denial of human rights. Shan threatens to go to the Governor to complain about the University's policies on freedom and democracy."

"What? I don't support any Chinese policies," Roger said.

Hamilton continued, "I called him as soon as his letter came in. His politics are way left of center, but that doesn't matter much. He says that by accepting a donor body, you caused a prisoner's death, probably a Uyghur. So, by receiving your transplant, you supported the Communist party's policies."

Roger asked, "And what am I to do? I can't return the body. The Chinese doctors told me that authorities condemned a prisoner to death for a crime. He chose to donate his body instead of being shot."

"We have to deal with Professor Shan. I've scheduled a meeting for you, me, Shan, and the University's human rights attorney today at 2 o'clock. I have no solutions at the moment. We don't want demonstrations and that kind of thing. The President has asked me to handle the matter. Can you make the meeting?"

"Absolutely. See you then." He was relieved to hear that he would confront Professor Shan so soon. "Marsha, cancel my afternoon to rearrange my schedule. We have to deal with the protest thing."

He had problems concentrating while he awaited his 2 o'clock meeting. Marsha, looking worried, insisted on fetching him a submarine sandwich, half of which he choked down with a Coke. He tried playing solitaire on his terminal.

He arrived at Stanley Hamilton's office five minutes before 2. An assistant ushered him into a small conference room holding two men. The Vice President, in shirtsleeves, rose to greet him with a handshake. "Hello, Doctor Scully. Let me introduce you to Bruce Ames. Bruce is the university's lawyer for human rights and that sort of thing. Shan should be here shortly." Roger shook the hand of the dark-suited Black man.

"I'm here mostly to listen to what Professor Shan is complaining about. I've had one other dealing with him, which I can't get into," Ames said.

At that point, a tall bearded man in a corduroy jacket with leather elbow patches entered the room. He exchanged curt nods with Ames, then turned his attention to Hamilton, who arose. "Professor Shan, I'm Stan Hamilton."

The newcomer appeared not to see Hamilton's extended hand but instead nodded and turned his gaze to Roger. "And this is Professor Scully. Thank you for coming, and please have a seat."

Shan was seated opposite Roger at the round table and stared at him with no facial expression.

Hamilton immediately turned to Shan. "Why don't you explain your concern to Mr. Ames and Professor Scully?"

"I teach a course called International Human Rights. It requires the previous completion of Sociology 101. During the fall semester, a few students approached me to discuss human rights in China. At first, they requested a course on this topic. I explained that setting up a new course would involve bureaucratic approval and cause considerable delay. I suggested an informal seminar, which I volunteered to lead. They accepted the idea, and when we announced the project, fourteen students signed on. We meet every Saturday for three hours.

"For some months, the plight of the Chinese Uyghurs has been a topic of discussion. Seminar participants read two books—*Larry's Kidney* and *The Red Market*. Those books detail the dirty business of selling organs in China, often to wealthy Americans. When the university announced appointing a recipient of a Chinese prisoner's body, my students were enraged. They believe that the University of Colorado should not support this Chinese business by hiring a product of Chinese transplanting. The major source of organs is the Uyghur people, who are being oppressed, sterilized, and killed off in great numbers for so-called crimes. On Saturday, some students decided to welcome Professor Scully to demonstrate their feelings."

Hamilton spoke first. "Who are these students?"

"I can supply you with a list of their names. The group debated the issue and decided to be transparent. About half the students are foreign, from Southeast Asia. The two from China fear reprisals when they return home, so I suggest not releasing their names to the press. The protest demonstration is not part of the seminar; that activity is an initiative of the students themselves."

Hamilton said, "Do I understand that you advocate firing Professor Scully because of his medical history?"

"I am not suggesting that, but my students think he should go."

Ames leaned forward and said, "Firing a tenured professor is a difficult process that normally would not occur because of student protest. No one is accusing Professor Scully of any wrongdoing before or after his hiring. President Smith was involved in recruiting

Doctor Scully. He suggests that a committee consider the matter."

"The usual academic solution to everything, appoint a committee," Shan said with a sneer. "Will my students participate?"

"And meanwhile, those students are outside my office trashing my reputation," Roger responded, his face flushed with anger.

"What reputation?" Shan shot back. "You've never taught before. You've barely worked as a transplant surgeon. Your donor's body earned you this position, nothing more."

Hamilton held up his hands. "Gentlemen, let's be calm about this. President Smith's suggestion is good. I'll meet with him to discuss the committee appointments. I'm sure there will be a student representative. In the meantime, I suggest that the students stop demonstrating. Professor Shan, can you arrange that?"

"I'll ask them, but I can't interfere with their first amendment rights. Representation on the committee will encourage their cooperation."

"Please expedite that request and call me back. Your students have made their point. Further harassment of Professor Scully won't help anything. Gentlemen, I'll get back to all of you after I've met with the President."

Hamilton stayed Roger's departure with a gesture. "I'm sorry to see your start here get mired in University politics. I'm sure it'll work out." On his return to the office, Roger noticed the demonstrators departing, led by Professor Shan.

He was barely back in his office, rearranging his schedule with Marsha, when Ruben Smith, the President, was on the line. "Look, Roger, I'm sorry about this protest. Give us a few weeks or months to deal with it. I'm calling for another reason. The Governor has invited you and me to dinner at the mansion Thursday night. Are you available?"

"Yes, of course. What's the occasion?"

"The Governor is keenly interested in your Institute and wants to hear about your plans. You'll meet a few other political types. Very casual. Can you make 7 p.m. at the mansion?"

"I look forward to it." Roger went off to his first re-scheduled appointment, Associate Dean Schneider.

Roger was highly impressed by meeting again with Jan Schneider, Administrative Dean. Jan was quick, blunt, and at the same time, helpful. "Before you joined your Institute and the department was still only an idea, we put a line item in the budget for $100,000 in the current academic year. Since there are only a few months left, you have lots of money to run on until June 1st. I need you to create a budget for your department for the next academic year. All of the other clinical departments have already submitted theirs, so you're starting from behind. You'll need salaries for new faculty and clerical staff and a fair amount of travel to cover your recruiting efforts. Show me a draft budget before you submit your final request.

Roger's meeting with Bill Mercer gave him a fresh appreciation of the problems for his new department. After renewing their acquaintance, Mercer observed, "Your new department has raised some concerns. A lot of people want to know if you are going to be doing transplants. The urologists already transplant kidneys, the cardiothoracic guys are doing lungs and hearts, and the orthopedic and plastic surgeons argue over hands. They haven't done any hand replacements yet. Plastic surgery and ENT (otolaryngology) are both interested in doing faces, although they haven't done any of those yet. There's a lot of optimism about transplant surgery, but no one seems to think it is a specialty unto itself. I suggest you work closely with the surgical subspecialties so they view you as an ally instead of a threat. You could start by offering cross-appointments in your new department to the people we already have. I suggest that when you have candidates for hiring, you run them past the appropriate subspecialty so they will get hospital privileges, which they'll need.

"You may find some jealousy from other departments in the medical school because of your Institute funding. When the Colorado Marijuana Industry Association announced its funding of the Institute, it meant you didn't have to compete for University money or grants in the same way as other departments. Enjoy your independence."

"Associate Dean Reiker and I had an interesting conversation about me. You know I had a corporeal transplant. Where does that fit in with your surgical subspecialties?" Roger asked.

"That's an interesting question. Since you're handling brains, the neurosurgeons would like to be involved, even if they've never done one. They're smart and generally have no conflict with other specialties except in back surgery, where they compete with the orthopedic surgeons. If there's a chance of getting into the business of corporeal transplants, I suggest you talk to Ian Turnbull, the head of neurosurgery. You might also meet with the cardiovascular surgeons because of the vascular issues in such transplants."

"Dr. Reiker suggested that my new Institute be better housed in with the basic sciences instead of clinical. Do you have any views on that?"

"I understand we're going to have a meeting about that. I have no strong feelings on the matter; I can see a rationale for either location."

When he returned to the office, Marsha said, "You've had two calls from media outlets wanting interviews about the protests. How do you want to handle it?"

"I'm not available to any of them."

"Then watch what you answer on your cell. They'll try to get at you."

By 5 p.m., Roger was mentally exhausted. He skipped the gym he intended to visit on the way back to the apartment, resolving to do that in the morning.

At 6 p.m., Lishan called him on WeChat. "Professor Osler and I spoke about the job you mentioned. Despite my reservations about moving to America, I agreed to fly to Denver in a few weeks for an interview. But now, President Trump has barred all Chinese from entering the country, so we had to postpone my trip."

"Lishan, I'm excited you are thinking of coming here. I'm sure this virus thing will be over in a few months or so. You still have more than three months to finish your residency. Travel should be no problem by then," Roger said.

"You don't understand. If your president can act like that so suddenly, where would that leave me if I had come home to visit my family? This is the kind of thing that makes me nervous. I'm going to fly to Xinhua for an interview in three weeks. We'll see what comes of Denver, but it looks unlikely."

"Aw, gee, I'm sorry. I had my hopes up that you would come and like the job and Denver and stay here. Don't give up on it just yet."

"I'm not ruling out Denver, but it doesn't look possible at the moment. Changing the subject, how was your first day in the new job?"

He elected not to mention the protests but briefly explained the bureaucracy, and Lishan had to sign off for an early morning scrub. *Why did this virus thing have to screw up everything?*

He turned on the TV for the Bruins hockey game. The preceding local newscast featured a clip of the protesters in front of his office.

Fortunately, returning to Denver after his Asian hiatus, he still had a coterie of friends from his previous stay. George and Marion Hill invited him for dinner. After hugs and handshakes, George said, "You warned us that your appearance had changed. You got that right. Are you all settled? How's the new job?"

"I was lucky to get an apartment in the same building as before and use all the stuff I had stored, so I moved in pretty easily. The University is another matter. I never understood the amount of bureaucracy involved, but I guess I'll learn. I finally found time to drop into the ER and see everyone there. They gave me a nice welcome. The new Director was my resident a few years ago, and it was nice to see him advancing. I felt at home to be back in the hospital."

George leaned forward. "Roger, we heard about you the day you spoke in Florida. We were stunned and tried to contact you but didn't have any luck. Besides all the surgical issues, what was it like to wake up in a different body?"

Roger responded, "Scary at first. Remember, I was coming out of a long coma, not knowing the reason for the surgery or the nature of the operation. I was confused, and then I suddenly saw myself in a mirror, with the wrong face! It was like a nightmare. When I finally knew what had happened and saw a picture of myself after the hemicorporectomy, I understood. It was also clear that there was no alternative donor; the only available donor was Chinese." They gasped when he showed them the picture of him post-hemicorporectomy.

"Tell us all about living in China," Marion suggested.

"Well, I wouldn't want to generalize because China is so big and diverse. Unfortunately, most of my time has been in Harbin, which is bleak, desolate, bitter cold, and with horrible air pollution. You wear a mask all the time you are outside because of the air quality. And the cuisine is more Russian than what we think of as Chinese. I got along there, but I could never feel at home in any sense."

After the couple had brought him up to date on Denver gossip and family changes, Roger spent the rest of the evening recounting his medical journey with the multiple surgeries, ending with the corporeal transplant. As a surgeon himself, George was intrigued by the technology of the surgery and had many questions. He would never have imagined moving a brain into another person's skull. Marion left that part of the conversation to get six-year-old Oscar off to bed.

Marion returned, and they retired to the living room for coffee and cognac. "Roger, why don't you come up to the cabin on Friday for some skiing this weekend? There's not much of the season remaining, but the corn snow is still great," Marion suggested.

With a big smile, Roger replied, "Sounds great, and I'll accept. You have to realize, though, that most of my skills left with my other body, and I didn't get much muscle memory from my donor." He recounted his recent struggles to regain his skiing ability.

"I never thought of that," nodded George. "You would have to get all your muscle memory back."

"My first post-op challenge was tying my shoelaces," Roger said as he described the many challenges of relearning routine movements. "I'll ski the easy runs this weekend. Don't expect me on the black diamond courses."

Marion looked concerned. "Roger, we didn't see much of you after Joanne died. We loved her so much. How are you feeling now about that?"

"I still miss her, but now I can talk about it. I was pretty depressed in the months after she died. It was one of the reasons I took the trip to Tibet, but so much has happened. I still get the blues when I think about our plans to have a family." He elected not to discuss Lishan with his friends.

Roger drove back to his apartment in a good mood. Renewing his previous friendships made him feel at home. However, the evening made him recall his earlier life in Denver when he and Joanne often shared dinners and ski weekends with George and Marion. Tonight he looked forward to the weekend at their cabin and the opportunity to bring his skiing abilities back to their previous level.

On Thursday night, as he drove to the mansion, Roger was curious, wondering why the governor would invite him. Was there a political reason or someone's curiosity to see and meet the man who had changed bodies? The door opened before he could knock or ring a bell.

"Good evening, Doctor Scully. I'm David Pinsky, on the Governor's staff." They shook hands. "Come along, and let me introduce you." Roger mused, *Asian face must be Dr. Scully.*

Pinsky led him to the reception room, simply furnished with the bar at one end. On the walls were a series of stunning photographs of Colorado scenes. Governor Lupen, tall and distinguished-looking, held a martini in his left hand while talking to two well-dressed gentlemen. At introductions, his handshake was warm and firm but not crushing.

"Welcome back to Denver, Doctor Scully. I hope you're getting settled in at the University. We have great hopes for your new Institute."

"It's great to be back, Governor. It's a distinct improvement over living in Harbin, China," Roger explained.

"Meet Peter Weaver, the President of the Marijuana Growers Association. Some of us call him Peter the Potter as a joke. But he's the man who led the campaign to make marijuana legal, as it should be. I would also like you to meet Michael Goodman, our Colorado Secretary of Commerce."

While exchanging handshakes, Roger watched the approach of a tall and slim blond woman in a simple but elegant black dress. Roger judged her to be under thirty years of age. Her right eyebrow arched upward; he could see a faint scar above it. In her left hand, she carried what appeared to be a martini. Roger noticed there was no wedding ring.

"Doctor Scully, let me introduce you to my daughter Jessica. I should explain that she is not here as my daughter but as my senior political consultant," said the Governor.

"It's my pleasure to meet you, Doctor Scully. I've heard a lot about you. But these men all have their cocktails; you have none. What can I get you?" she said with a smile.

"Manhattan, straight up if you please," Roger answered. Moments later, she returned with his cocktail.

"Let me introduce you to any of the others you don't already know," she offered. "I understand you know the University President and the Vice President of Health Sciences. The gentleman over there talking to Doctor Smith is Bernard Weitzel, our Attorney General. Do you know him?"

When Roger indicated he did not, she gently guided him by the elbow across the room to the two men and made the introduction to Weitzel. Roger also shook hands with the University President. Smith explained to Weitzel that Roger had previously been in Denver as the director of the ER at the University hospital but was originally from Boston.

"So, what brought you to Denver originally?" Weitzel asked.

"Well, it was a good job offer for me, and one for my late wife, and at least as important, the mountains for the hiking and skiing," Roger replied with a slight frown as he remembered Joanne.

At that point, David Pinsky made a loud clap with his hands and announced they should take their places for dinner in the adjoining dining room. Roger noticed the table set for eight with the Governor at one end, the Attorney General at the other. Roger was pleased that his place card put him between Weaver and Jessica. Roger detected a faint floral rose scent from her, similar to Joanne's *Miss Dior*.

"Folks, thank you all for coming. We will discuss a little business after dinner. In the meantime, you'll all enjoy the home cooking here at the mansion," said the Governor.

As the waiter poured the wine, Jessica turned to him and said, "I heard about your problem with protesters this week."

"No problem, but I'd rather discuss something more pleasant."

"Agreed, so tell me about your skiing. Where are you skiing now?"

He did not ask her how she knew he was a skier. Roger replied that he had done almost no challenging skiing recently but was planning on going to Loveland in a few days. He explained the difficulty of regaining his skiing skills earlier in the year.

She nodded her understanding. "Loveland is a good choice for all levels of skills. Our family has had a cabin there since I was a child. I might see you there. Are you going this weekend, Dr. Scully?"

"Yes," he answered. I'm staying with the Hills, who own a cabin there. But call me Roger."

"I read the University's press release about your appointment. You're one of the most interesting people I've ever met. How about your family? I know you lost your wife a while back. Do you have children?"

"No kids. How did you know about my wife?"

"I'll let you in on something. For security reasons, we do a background check on anyone visiting the mansion. I peeked at your file before you came. Let's get back to skiing."

He found it a bit creepy to have someone do a background check before a dinner invite. *I can imagine this in China, but in America?* When he inquired about her skiing experience, Jessica replied, "As an undergraduate, I was on the Dartmouth ski team and tried out for the national and Olympic team for the downhill. I came close, but I wasn't up to the level of those doing it full-time. A serious fall almost ended my career. That's the scar over my eye. But it was a good experience. I had also decided that law school was more important than skiing."

"Where did you do law school?"

"Harvard."

"Where do you practice?" Roger asked.

"Not yet. I came here directly from law school to help my dad and take the bar exam. I passed it last month. Because it's an election year, I've agreed to stay on here until November. Then I'll get a real job. I'm talking to a few firms here and in Boulder, but I haven't made any decisions yet."

"Are you going to stay in politics?"

"Hell, NO. I've grown up with politics, lived and breathed politics, and I've had enough of politics. Do you realize this is my fourth dinner out this week for my dad? I love him dearly, but I want to settle down and be away from politics as soon as the election is over."

She changed the subject. "Did you say you're skiing Loveland this weekend?"

"Yeah, but I'm going to have to arrange some lessons. Remember I told you about having to regain muscle memory."

"Let me make a suggestion. One of my old boyfriends is the best instructor around. He's a very well-educated ski bum—Loveland in our winter, Chile in our summer. When we've finished dinner, I can make a call if you like. I'm going to be at Loveland this weekend. Saturday night, I'll be having dinner at The Bistro with two girlfriends of mine. Care to join us?"

"Sure, sounds like fun. I'm staying with friends, so can I catch a ride for dinner?" Jessica and Roger made their ride arrangements.

As dessert dishes were disappearing, the governor stood up. "Thank you all for coming. Consider this as the informal celebration of the start of the Life Prolongation Institute. We are fortunate to have here tonight the new director, Roger Scully. Roger, I should have warned you before you came, but could you please give us a short explanation of the mission of your Institute?"

Roger stood up. "The title says it all, Life Prolongation. Specifically, we intend to use organ transplants and new technologies to replace or assist organs. Everyone here is familiar with kidney transplants, and you have all heard about my whole-body transplant. Unfortunately, there's a worldwide shortage of organs for people in desperate need of them. We need to use various solutions—animal organs, artificial organs, and human donors. Most of you probably know someone with an aortic valve replacement. In all likelihood, that valve came from a pig. The artificial heart is now a functioning device but not perfect enough for prolonged use. Human donors are usually the best, but there are too few of them. Some scientists are growing brain tissue that may be used to replace damaged or missing parts of the brain.

"I'm famous or infamous for suggesting that prisoners be allowed to donate blood or other organs. We're failing our dying patients because we have not yet established a functioning system of organ donation. I would hope, Governor, that Colorado could again show some leadership by making it possible for prisoners to donate blood or organs.

"Meanwhile, my institute will work on perfecting animal transplants and developing technologies that will reduce the need for human transplants. I'm grateful to Mr. Weaver and his industry for giving me this opportunity. I'll try not to disappoint you." Nodding to the table, he resumed his seat.

"Isn't there a law against prisoners donating organs?" asked the Governor.

Roger replied, "Your daughter or Attorney General might correct me, sir, but I am aware of no state or federal law that prohibits prisoners from donating blood or organs. It's a problem with state and federal corrections departments that don't allow it."

Jessica spoke up. "Doctor Scully is correct. There is no law against it."

The Governor looked concerned. "Jessica, please get me more information on this policy. I want to do the right thing."

Peter Weaver spoke up, "My colleagues and I are delighted that we have a director who is a visionary with the leadership qualities to make a difference. Good luck to you, Doctor Scully." He raised his wine glass in a toast to Roger.

As the table broke up from dinner, Jessica was making a call. "Hello Allen, it's your old buddy, Jessica again—yes, I'm fine, but I need a favor this weekend." She went on to explain Roger's need for ski lessons. Looking over at Roger, she asked, "Allen says he can give you a private lesson this Saturday from 9 until 12. Okay?" When Roger smiled and nodded, she returned to the call. "Great, Allen. Thanks, and see you soon."

Home relatively early, he reflected on his first week in the new position. *I've got a great job. I'm back with old friends. I just met an attractive and smart woman. Life is looking good, and now I'm Roger Scully, full-time.* But the same nagging concern, *Am I up to the job?*

CHAPTER 20

Roger was excited and primed for the Friday trip to familiar Loveland. He was with old friends, looked forward to skiing, and anticipated another meeting with Jessica. As promised, he had picked up three prime porterhouse steaks and a bottle of excellent red zin. Marion had agreed to supply vegetables and salad. While waiting for their partially-prebaked potatoes to finish, Roger marinated the steaks as the group enjoyed their usual pre-dinner cocktails.

Roger opened the conversation. "It feels great to be back here with you folks. The only thing missing is Joanne."

"We miss her, too," said Marion, with a wistful smile. "But you have a new life now. You mentioned you have a date for tomorrow night. Who's the lucky woman?"

"I'm not sure you call it a date. Jessica Lupen, she's the Governor's daughter. I had dinner at the mansion earlier in the week and sat next to her. We got talking skiing, and she arranged a lesson for me tomorrow with her ex-boyfriend and then suggested I join her with two of her girlfriends at The Bistro."

George flashed a wide grin. "Well, start at the top and have three women at your table. Sounds great. I'm glad to see you're back in circulation."

"She must be a lot better skier than me. She tried out for the Olympic team, and she's going cat skiing tomorrow. I tried it a few times before and loved it, but I have to do some more work on my skills before I trust myself on some of those runs."

"What took you to the Governor's mansion?" Marion asked.

"The Governor is interested in my new Institute. He arranged the dinner to introduce me to Peter Weaver, the CEO of the Marijuana Growers Trade Association. I think I told you before that they're funding the Life Prolongation Institute." Dinner conversation turned to politics but ended early. They planned to make an early start the next day.

Saturday morning, Roger was pleased with his guide, Allen, a lean and bearded man with a chronic sunburn. After handshakes, he said, "Okay, Roger. Why don't I give you a tryout on the intermediate slope, and then we'll see what you need from me." The Poma lift took them to the top of a mogul-infested, moderately inclined, well-packed run. Allen pointed out the course and explained he would follow Roger to watch his performance.

At the bottom of the slope, he nodded approval. "I think you can handle something more challenging. You seem to know what you're doing. Why did you have Jessica arrange a lesson?"

Roger paused and decided to lie a little, "I've been off skis for some time due to health reasons. I thought it wise to get checked out by someone competent before I tried serious slopes."

They mounted the chairlift. The bright sun, cool breeze, and gentle sway hypnotized Roger on the chair. He almost fell asleep.

"I haven't seen Jessica for months. How's she doing?" Allen asked.

"She's well, and I'll see her tonight for dinner. I think she's a tad tired of politics. She wants to find another job after the election. She called you her ex-boyfriend. Was she correct?"

"Oh, yeah. Mild scandal. Everyone knows we went to Chile to ski one summer. We had a blast but decided a long-term relationship was not a great idea. We're still friends, but I rarely see her. You're probably more her type since you have a real career." Roger closed his eyes for the few minutes of the ride remaining.

The downhill run ran rapidly with the smooth swish sounds interspersed with the slap of tails coming off a snowy hump. Twice Roger threatened to tumble but caught himself while his heart pounded. The thrills were back; Roger had returned. By noon he felt younger than his thirty-nine years, healthier, and in control of not just his skills but his life. His guide, Allen, met him at the bottom. "Congratulations, Roger. You can handle any run on this mountain, including the cat routes. Go and enjoy! That applies to skiing **and** Jessica."

He met George and Marion for a patio lunch. Marion observed, "Roger, I don't know if it's the sun, the wind, or your attitude. Your face is glowing."

Roger answered with a smile. "It's great to be back on the mountain in the sun. I've recovered most of my skiing skills. I'm with friends that I love. I have a challenging job. And best of all, I'm back in the U.S.A., as the Boss would say."

They toasted him with their coffee cups, and all agreed to finish skiing at 3 p.m. On his next run, he lost an edge, fell hard, and followed with a long slide. Uninjured, he stood up, brushed off the snow, and decided to dial back his aggressive approach.

At 6:45, Jessica picked him up at the cabin. Roger nodded approvingly when she drove up in her green Range Rover. After exchanging greetings, Jessica asked, "How was your lesson today?"

"I was happy. Mostly, Allen just watched. At the end of the lesson, he said I could do any of the runs, including cat skiing. Maybe next week, I'll sign up for a day."

"You'll be lucky if the snow quality holds. We'll see. Here's The Bistro."

The hostess recognized Jessica as they entered, greeted her by name, and hugged her briefly. Roger decided Jessica was a regular here. On the way to the table, Marlene, one of their dinner party, intercepted them, and Jessica introduced her. When they arrived at the table, Marlene said, "Roger, meet my wife, Norma."

Roger was embarrassed that his startled look betrayed his surprise. Jessica laughed and said, "Relax, Roger, they're queer, but I'm very straight." He interpreted that remark as designed to keep him interested in furthering a relationship. She continued, "Let's get the rules straight. Separate checks for Roger and me. I'm limited to one glass of wine because the Governor's daughter dares not commit DUI."

The dinner proceeded in a light-hearted fashion. Near the end of the meal, Marlene raised her glass. "Here's to Roger: welcome back to the USA. What's it like to be home?"

Roger replied, "At times in China, I felt I was living in a spy movie. I was working as a surgeon, living with a Chinese woman doctor, and feeling less and less comfortable. I was lucky to land my job in Denver. I have no intention to return to China." He did not mention his dual citizenship.

"And where in China were you?" asked Marlene.

"Mostly in Harbin, in the northeast, near the Russian border. It has nasty cold winters aggravated by horrible air pollution. The food has a distinct Russian influence, which doesn't improve things."

Marlene continued, "I would have to say that you don't look very Chinese. You have beautiful round eyes in a handsome face. Your body looks fit. If I was into men, I could go for you!" The two women looked at Jessica, who blushed slightly, to Roger's delight.

Jessica was driving him back to his friend's cabin. "I'm not skiing tomorrow. My dad has yet another dinner function I have to attend. What are your plans for next weekend?"

"I don't have any. My friends won't be up here, but I can use their cabin."

"We don't know how much longer the snow will last. Next weekend may be it. Can I invite you to ride with me to stay in my cabin next Friday?"

"Sounds great. What can I bring?"

"You can bring the food for breakfast Saturday and Sunday morning, and I'll prepare the Friday dinner with steak."

"And I'll bring a decent cabernet to go with it." They had arrived at the cabin. "Thank you for a great evening. Your friends were good company, the food was excellent, and you are charming. Can I kiss you goodnight?" He leaned over the center compartment. Her open-mouth kiss was not the perfunctory peck he expected. That seems like a promise! His feet fairly floated over the skiffle of snow on the walk to the cabin door.

Monday morning found Roger in the office before 8, refreshed and renewed. He was on his desk computer when Marsha entered. "You've got some color in your cheeks, Boss. How was the skiing?"

"Great. I need to add another appointment for this week. Do you know Brenda Gillespie, the Chair of Genetics?"

"I know of her but never met her personally."

"There's several things I would like to discuss. See if you can get me an appointment this week."

Thirty minutes later, Marsha said, "Dr. Gillespie suggests coffee at her office tomorrow at 10. Your calendar's clear. Shall I accept?"

"Please. And then let's get working on this damn budget." They spent the rest of the day finishing a draft budget. Marsha was a great assistant since she had been through the process before.

Tuesday morning, Roger approached the Department of Human Genetics with some anxiety. Aside from his departmental concerns, he intended to raise some personal issues. Brenda Gillespie was an imposing much-published authority in her field. After pleasantries regarding his appointment and objectives for the Institute, she asked, "How can my department help you in your rather daunting endeavor?"

"Some of what we do will be at the intersection of surgery, genetics, and immunology. Beyond DNA typing to match organ donors to patients, there is the issue of whether the transplant alters the genetic makeup of the recipient."

Dr. Gillespie raised her eyebrows in an unspoken question. Roger continued, "As you know, a person with a transplant is technically a chimera, having DNA from two sources. Since my transplant, I'm a chimera." She nodded her understanding. "I've now come across a couple of papers suggesting that, say a kidney transplant, shows up as a second type of DNA in a cheek swab or a semen sample. Are you familiar with that work?"

"Yes, we try to avoid the field, but the forensic geneticists are having hissy fits over a couple of cases. One man was arrested for rape when his DNA in the FBI database created a match. He proved he was a few thousand miles away at the time of the rape. His kidney donor was the guilty party, but it took a lot of legal work to get through HIPPA restrictions. And then, in some sheriff's lab, one of their own had his sperm DNA change after a marrow transplant. As far as I know, no one has come up with an explanation for the phenomenon. It contradicts what we thought we understood about DNA behavior. Since the FBI has DNA profiles of more than a million people, there's an opportunity for serious mischief."

"We've been reading the same reports. Now Brenda, from all the publicity, you know that I am a chimera. I've been assuming I could not pass on my original genes since I have my donor's testes. Is it possible that my sperm might contain Scully genes instead of the genes of my donor?" Roger asked.

"You ask an interesting and appropriate question. I'm afraid I don't have an answer. If you like, we can do your DNA profile, perhaps blood, saliva, and sperm. It may satisfy your curiosity, but I'm not sure what you do with the information. For instance, you might think you can select the spermatocyte for an intended pregnancy through in-vitro fertilization. Because of CRISPR, it is theoretically possible to alter an ovum or sperm cell to obliterate or change certain genes. Most of us in the field, including me, consider this an unethical use of our technology. I sum it up by telling my students, 'Don't monkey with the gametes!' Do you get what I mean?"

"I think I understand you. I'd still like to know more about my genetic makeup. It may be more complicated because, before the brain transplant, the surgical team replaced the donor's marrow with mine to minimize rejection phenomena."

"Wow, you are interesting. A donation from a chimera to create another chimera. We'll be most interested in investigating your DNA if you don't mind being some kind of one-person study in human biology."

"I'm quite used to being the specimen under the microscope."

After a short discussion concerning the need for confidentiality, Brenda called in her most senior technician, who scheduled specimen collection, including a fresh sperm sample, for the following day. Roger left, understanding that he could expect results about ten days later, at which time Brenda would discuss them.

Friday found Roger distracted from his university duties, excited for the weekend. With his late afternoon committee meeting canceled, he left the office before 3. He picked up eggs, thinly sliced prosciutto, sourdough bread, shredded cheddar cheese, porcini mushrooms, butter, and fresh cilantro at the supermarket. He also added a reasonably priced bottle of champagne and a more expensive cabernet. Roger dropped a box of condoms into his grocery order. He was planning his weekend.

At 4:30 p.m., when Jessica pulled up in front of the apartment building, Roger was leaning against a tree, smiling. On the ground beside him were his skis and poles, boots, a duffel bag, and a large cooler. Out of the car, she strode over to him, put her right hand on his left shoulder, and kissed his cheek, startling him. Roger decided she looked as attractive in jeans and sneakers as in her more formal attire.

"You're traveling light these days," Jessica laughed.

"Well, you did give me the responsibility for breakfast, and this is the only cooler I own." He nodded to the large Yeti cooler.

"I look forward to your cooking," she said.

While Jessica clamped his skis to her roof rack, Roger loaded everything else into the Range Rover. He felt a rush of enthusiasm as she started the drive to the mountain. He felt very comfortable in her presence but also detected in himself a hormonal surge. Jessica turned off the car radio, indicating a desire for conversation.

"Do you have any brothers or sisters?" Roger asked.

"I have a younger brother Pete, a sophomore at Dartmouth."

"You must've liked the place to recommend it to him. Is he a competitive skier too?"

"Nah, he prefers snowboarding. He tried competing a few years ago but lost interest. He enjoys the sport, but he's never been as competitive as I am."

"That's interesting. What else do you compete in?" Roger asked as he watched her face.

"Well, maybe competitive is the wrong term. I don't compete against other people as much as I enjoy challenging myself. I did very well in college but was never trying to beat others. I am one of those weirdos who loves taking exams. Each one is a challenge. Flyfishing is the same way; every cast, every stream, and every day is different. There is always room for improvement, which makes me a little humble even when I make a great cast."

"I can understand that," Roger nodded.

"To be a good lawyer, you should be self-confident but always aware of your weaknesses. And what about you? Getting into med school is one of the most competitive things I can imagine. What else do you compete in?"

"You're right about the competition for med school. Between the pre-med requirements, which are heavy subjects with laboratories, and realizing that 80 percent or more of your classmates will not get accepted into med school, it doesn't lead to much camaraderie or fun. I played hockey in high school and enjoyed it. In college and med school, I played intramurals. In Denver before, I played in a midnight league of old men like me and even older. We played women's rules, with no body-checking. It's safer but takes some of the fun out of the game. I may go back to it next year."

Jessica frowned, "What makes my head spin is that you sound like an American straight out of Boston, and yet, you're, uh, Chinese. It's not a problem and nothing against you. I'm sorry, I must sound like a horrible racist, but I'm not. Forgive me if I upset you."

With a smile, Roger replied, "No, I feel better that we can have this discussion openly. Once in a while, I find myself doing a double-take in the mirror, asking, "Is that me? Do you know I have a Chinese name?"

"Oh, you have an actual Chinese name?"

"Yeah. It's a long story, and I'd rather tell it over a drink. We'll deal with it later. Let's change the subject for now."

"We'll discuss dinner. I suggest we cook dinner at my place tonight; we can eat at a restaurant tomorrow. I have a lovely slab of tenderloin and everything for salad. Do you like bison? My uncle's ranch keeps us supplied."

"How cool is that. I only had it once before, and I enjoyed it. I understand that it's healthier than beef. Your dinner idea sounds good to me."

Jessica described the Denver apartment she had closed on earlier in the day. "My cottage at the Governor's mansion was okay, but it was a little weird," she said. "No privacy at all, with everyone having to go in and out through security. I'll cook my food on my own, thank you. I took two bedrooms because I like to have a proper home office. At least in Denver, we don't have the atrocious rents of San Francisco or New York."

"I did the same thing, taking two bedrooms. I have my desk and elliptical trainer in the spare room. When I lived here before, we were looking at houses and planning a family. That seems a long way back now, but I'll probably start looking at houses again in a few months. I want a garage with a workshop."

They were now in Loveland and approaching a security gate, which opened when the car was about ten feet away. Seeing the surprised look on Roger's face, Jessica explained, "There's some kind of magnetic strip on my car that the machine recognizes. I'm not a big fan of gated communities; I think it is a bit snobbish. My grandad bought the cottage for my twenty-first birthday. It was sort of a consolation prize, I guess. Team USA for the Olympics had just cut me, and Grandad wanted to cheer me up, which he did. Loveland has always been my home turf for skiing. In the summer, there's challenging hiking and a few trout streams nearby."

They arrived at a rather ordinary-looking single-story house. The driveway to the attached garage was bare of snow, while the landscape's remainder was snow-covered. "Who shovels your drive?" Roger asked.

"Nobody. The driveway has electric cables in it that automatically melt the snow and ice for me. It means I can arrive without having to shovel my way to the house." The wide garage door swung up at the push of a dashboard button. Once inside, Roger noted four pairs of skis on racks and several fly rod tubes. A six-foot workbench and a covered barbeque also drew his interest. "I suggest you leave your skis on my car till you need them tomorrow."

From the garage, they entered through a laundry/utility room to a traditional kitchen. The gas range had four burners and a grill, with two ovens underneath and a large stainless steel hood over the top. A sub-zero refrigerator and similar freezer stood against the sidewall. The glass door showed the freezer to be almost full.

"Wow, are you planning to cook for a lot of people?" Roger asked.

"Hey, I'm from a Mormon family, and food ahead is always there. Bring your gear along here," she said as she trundled her small case through a large room with a fireplace, sofa, easy chairs, and a dining set of a table with six chairs. They entered a hallway. At the first pair of opposing doors, she gestured to the right and said, "That's your room. I hope it's okay. You'll find the hot water takes forever to reach you. I'll see you in the kitchen in a few minutes." She entered the door opposite and closed it behind her.

He felt a slight disappointment. *I guess we're not sharing a bedroom tonight.* He unpacked his shaving kit, washed his hands and face, and brushed his hair before joining her in the kitchen. Her slim jeans emphasized her athletic body.

"I brought all the ingredients for the Black Manhattans I saw you order last week. I even found the right cherries, so I'll leave you to fix drinks while I fire up the grill in the garage. By the way, how do you like your steak?"

"Medium rare, but I'm not fussy. You're in charge here," replied Roger.

"Glad you understand that!" she laughed as she slid her hand over his buttocks, exiting the kitchen. *Is she coming on to me?* With a grin on his face, Roger quickly found a cocktail shaker and appropriate glasses. As he began shaking the mixture, Jessica reappeared with a plate. On that plate was a slice of bison tenderloin, an inch and half thick, covered in a reddish rub. Roger estimated the slab was well over one and a half pounds. Into each glass, he carefully dropped a Luxardo cherry from the Ziploc bag she had brought, then carefully sliced a small wedge of a navel orange. He drained the shaker into the two glasses.

"That's a pretty sight," Jessica said as she lifted her glass to his. "I think you have me hooked on these already."

"To a nice evening, a fun weekend, and happy times," echoed Roger as their eyes met over the glass rims. Roger hoped he was looking at a future relationship. They sat together on a small sofa with their drinks on the coffee table in front of them.

"Do you mind if we watch PBS news?" asked Jessica. I usually watch Friday nights because I like Brooks and Capehart."

"It suits me. Brooks is one of the few Republicans who makes sense. I assume that you're a Democrat?"

"Pretty easy assumption when my father is the Democratic Governor of the state. I have several Republican friends who can't stand our current president. When I'm with them, we don't discuss politics. Leaving politics, where are you skiing tomorrow?"

Roger replied, "Nothing planned. I called to ask about cat skiing to get into the backcountry, but they said it was finished for the season. Can you suggest something interesting but not too challenging since I'm still getting back my skills?"

"I'll show you a few good runs. I can't imagine what it must be like to do something that your brain finds familiar but your body finds new. I wonder how I would ski if I had a different body. I get confused just thinking about it. You must be a genius."

"Thank you, but I'm not. It's interesting, though, that the one thing that improved after my transplant was using chopsticks. I thought I was pretty good while I was waiting those months for the surgery, but my hands seemed to work more naturally afterward. Maybe I imagined it."

"Why did you have to wait months for the surgery?"

"You can't imagine the preparation. Here's what I looked like." He showed her the hemicorporectomy picture.

"Jesus Christ, I never imagined a person could look like that."

"Now you know why I needed the transplant. It took time to prepare my body, find a donor, and then prepare the donor."

"Who was the donor?" Jessica asked.

"A prisoner they'd condemned to death, for whatever crime. Would you believe that China has forty-six capital crimes? They sometimes give the condemned man a choice. Die under an anesthetic to donate your organs or be shot in the head. They consider that to be informed consent."

"I never knew about that part of your story. You have an unbelievable past. I get shivers thinking about it. And look at you now!"

"I'm happy with the outcome. I've got my life back. I'm over the nightmare."

She reached across his chest, grasped his right shoulder, and hugged him. "Thank you for sharing your story. I admire your courage to get through all that. You deserve some fun in your life. Let's do that together." She kissed him on the lips.

"Sounds good to me." Roger felt a warm rush of encouragement, an attraction beyond animal lust.

As Brooks and Capehart were finishing their TV dialogue, the Manhattan glasses were running dry. Jessica stood up, ate the entire orange slice in two bites, then poured the cherry into her mouth. "Let's make some dinner. The charcoal should be ready," she said as she returned to the kitchen, picked up the bison plate, and headed for the garage. Roger quickly returned to his room and reappeared to meet her with a 2010 bottle of Heitz cabernet sauvignon.

"This should go nicely," he grinned. "Where do you keep your corkscrew?"

Jessica nodded approval at the wine selection, opened a drawer, and handed him a corkscrew. "You can set the table while I fix the salad," she said as she slid a baguette into the oven. Meat, salad, and garlic bread are on the menu tonight." She rubbed a large wooden bowl with a cut garlic clove, then added balsamic vinegar, extra-virgin olive oil, and a few white anchovies from a jar. After mashing them in the oil and vinegar mixture, she used her large chef's knife to chop a romaine head that she tossed into the bowl. From the refrigerator, she drew a container of shaved parmesan, which she added to the lettuce. She deftly tossed the salad mixture with two wooden forks. "Done," she said. "The steak should be ready to turn." She headed for the garage door as Roger poured himself a taste of the cabernet. It swirled beautifully in the oversize wine glass. He nodded after he took a mouthful, rinsed it around in his mouth, then swallowed.

"Perfection," he whispered as he took the bottle and glasses to the dining table. A minute later, Jessica, back in the kitchen, fetched the baguette from the oven. She split it with her knife, then spread it with garlic butter she had prepared in advance. *She knows her way around the kitchen.* A moment later, she returned to the garage, emerging seconds later with the steak on the plate.

"Mmm, that looks and smells good," said Roger. She deftly carved the steaming steak on the cutting board to reveal a dark crust and moist pink interior for each slice. She divided the meat into two portions that she placed on two plates warming in the oven with the bread. Food in hand, they proceeded to the table.

Jessica tasted the wine, then reached for the bottle, which she inspected. "That's a famous label. I'm not used to drinking wine this old."

"Almost everyone drinks cabs that are too young. If you want something recent, stick to merlot or pinot noir. Most cabs are best when they're at least eight or ten years old."

"I didn't know that. So your taste memories didn't change when you swapped bodies?"

"Interesting point. Most taste comes from receptors in the nose, with the signal sent to the brain to interpret. The receptors are pretty much the same from person to person, but the interpretation remains in my original brain. Right after the transplant, I had no taste or smell until the nerves reconnected from my nose and throat to my brain. My brain recognizes the signal as taste or smell. It's complicated. I'm glad I have those senses back; this food is delicious."

"You promised to tell me about your Chinese name," Jessica reminded as they continued eating and drinking.

"Wu Zicheng." Roger explained his long wait in the hospital under his new name created to disguise his true identity. After the surgery, he needed to renew his passport and visa. He summarized his Chinese citizenship attainment, ending with, "I didn't have to give up my U.S.

passport to become Chinese. And there is no documentation in either country concerning my alternate identity."

"Fascinating," said Jessica with raised eyebrows. "You really are two persons with one body. I've never met anyone with such an unusual background."

"Outside of my parents, you are the only person in the country that knows my entire story, so I trust you to keep it confidential."

Roger reached over and started to replenish their wine glasses. Jessica smiled and said, "Whoa, boy. You don't need to get me drunk to fuck me."

Roger responded with a startled smile.

"Don't act so surprised. I'm sure you assumed when I invited you here that we would end up in bed. Am I a little too blunt? I've been lusting after you ever since we met for the first time at that dinner."

Roger answered, "Uh, surprised, yes, shocked, no, I appreciate your candor. It's great. I admit to my lust, but I was afraid I was rushing it." He now had his hand under her sweater, feeling firm breasts unconstrained by any brassiere. His fingers found the erect nipples. His mouth was at her neck, then at her open lips. Her hands were undoing his belt buckle.

She pulled her head back. "We're going to knock over the wine glasses. Let's move to my bedroom."

Roger half-stumbled to her bedroom, clutching at the top of his now-unfastened jeans to prevent them from falling past his slim hips. "I have some condoms in my duffle bag," he said.

"Maybe you can forget them. I have an IUD and no sex partners for months. What's your recent history?"

"Just the doctor I was living with. Monogamous."

"Then you can forget the condom."

Beside the bed, she dropped to her knees and pulled his jeans and shorts down. "Oh, look what I've found! Let me taste it."

His hands were clasped behind her head when she suddenly withdrew. "Let's get into bed before you fall over your jeans." In her bedroom, she pulled off her sweater and stepped out of her jeans and panties. He was stepping out of his clothes and doffing his polo shirt.

He stared at her. "Jessica, you are a woman of incredible beauty. You should never wear clothes."

Two hours later, they lay together, staring at the ceiling, both exhausted. Neither was thinking about skiing.

"I haven't been with that many men, but you are the best. I came at least three times."

"That's the advantage of older men. Women have taught them what to do. Am I sleeping here or in the other room?"

"I want you here, but I need a towel to deal with the wet spot under me."

"What? Did I do that?"

"We both contributed." When she returned with a small towel, they exchanged kisses and fell asleep in a spoon position.

At 7 a.m., she was aware that Roger was awake. She nudged his arm with her elbow. "Good morning, stud. Listen to that rain. Skiing just ended for the year. We'll have to think of something else to do today."

"I have a suggestion if I have another few hours of recovery."

"You're insatiable, which I like."

"Do you play, Go?" Roger asked.

"No, isn't that some oriental game played only by geniuses?"

"So, you qualify! I brought my portable game. We can have fun while we both learn. I'm still a long way from being a good player. Did you ever read the novel *Shibumi*?"

"Never heard of it," said Jessica, shaking her head.

"It's a cult classic, with a Go-Master who takes years to study the game. It's an erotic novel filled with evil plots and assassination. Wicked. It gave me fantasies when I read it."

"I'll take your word for it. I'll try to learn Go if you move your ass and cook our breakfast."

"I'll make your coffee to keep you occupied while I shower and cook."

As he prepared the breakfast, he reviewed his situation. *Jessica combines the best of Joanne and Lishan. I think I've lucked out.* Thirty minutes later, the table showed a prosciutto-porcini-cilantro omelet accompanied by mimosas.

Jessica appeared and viewed the spread. "I didn't know we had champagne for mimosas."

"One of my surprises, dear lady."

"You're full of surprises, all of them good so far. The omelet is delicious. Is cooking another of your talents?"

Following breakfast, they agreed that the continuing rain had ruined any hope of skiing for the weekend. Roger brought out his folding Go board and two bags of tiles. "If you have two small bowls, it'll make things easier. And a pencil and paper."

An hour later, Jessica sighed. "Roger, this game is impossible. I'll never be able to understand the scoring, let alone any strategy. You better find someone smarter."

"I'm sure you're smart enough, but finding playing partners is difficult."

As Roger packed up his game, Jessica went into the kitchen and returned with a plate of brownies and two mugs of coffee. "These are my special brownies. Completely legal, but pretty heavy with THC."

"Ah, the joys of being home. The Chinese have a curious relationship with marijuana. It's officially banned, but not much enforced. The Taoists have used it for centuries in their religious ceremonies and seem to get away with it. I didn't use any while I was away."

"Do you smoke or vape?" Jessica asked.

"Never. There's pretty good evidence that vaping or smoking pot can lead to lung damage. The THC effects are quicker than your brownies, but I don't like the idea of the risk. I smoked pot before med school but decided only to ingest it in the future. And your brownies are great."

Jessica asked, "How do you want to spend the rest of the weekend? Skiing is finished, likely for the season. The rain will make the road miserable for the rest of the day. We have enough food in the freezer for at least a month. There's no need to eat out."

"I feel like a bowl of soup. Pot always makes me hungry." He felt strongly attracted to her. *Is there a future here?* "I want to hear more about you. You know all about me, from the publicity. And then you read my background check, to which I officially object. Do you mind?"

"Fine with me. Soup will be on in a few minutes." Over the soup and remains of the baguette, Jessica started. "Third-generation Colorado, starting with Grandad's ranch, which my uncle now runs. Hence, the bison. You know my dad is a lawyer, a plaintiff's litigator always active in politics. Mom was stay-at-home, involved in volunteer work. You know, the usual symphony and art gallery boards locally. She was also on the Sierra Club national board. I went to public schools until I went off to Dartmouth. After that, Harvard law school."

"And the skiing?"

"Our family has always skied. I had my first pair of skis at age four and never looked back. I was competing nationally in high school. I had hoped for the Olympics but wasn't quite good enough. Skiing gave me a lot of travel, a lot of fun, and got me into Dartmouth."

"I thought the Ivy League didn't give athletic scholarships."

"They don't. But if you make the academic requirements in terms of GPA and SAT scores, they give the ski coach a certain number of men and women to pick from the qualified group. Since they only admit a fraction of those applicants meeting the scholastic requirements, jocks have an advantage. There was no money attached to it. I was lucky that my dad has done very well."

"What was your undergraduate major?" he asked.

"Biology. At one point, I almost went for a Ph.D. in wildlife biology."

"Cool. Did my background check show that my hobby is nature photography?"

"What a coincidence."

"Come see me sometime, and I'll show you my etchings."

"That's a different pick-up line. I'll be there."

"One of the reasons I was in Tibet when I was injured was a trek with the opportunity to spot and photograph a snow leopard. I'd still like to do that."

"Exciting. Can I come along?"

They spent the next three hours reviewing their camping, hiking, and climbing histories. By dinner time, they agreed that Roger needed to learn to fly fish, and Jessica would teach him. The dessert of Jessica's brownies gave them both a warm glow and a considerable release of inhibitions. Roger suggested, "You said you never read the novel *Shibumi,* but there was a game mentioned that I would like to try."

"Another version of Go?"

"No, listen to this. We each get out of our clothes and into robes. We sit cross-legged on the floor in front of the fire. Then we take turns. Each person has two minutes to do something sexy to excite the other. The only rule is no touching the other. You can say anything or do anything."

"And how do you win or lose?"

"Winner is the first one to bring the other to orgasm," Roger grinned.

"How many times have you played this game?"

"Never, but I've often thought about it."

The second and third brownies were taking effect. With a smile, Jessica said, "You're on, buddy. Let's move the coffee table to make some room here in front of the fireplace."

Two minutes later, they had moved the table and changed into their terrycloth robes. Sitting in front of the fire, Jessica said, "We'll use my watch with its timer. And you can go first."

In the years since he had read the book, he had, on occasion, contemplated a strategy. Self-control was paramount; defense took priority over offensive actions. For his first turn, he elected to use only his voice. "Your face is flushing a bit. Your nipples are getting hard and erect. You are watching my dick and hoping to see some change. You're starting to get a little wet. Your turn."

Jessica rose, stood two feet in front of him, and started a slow dance, accentuating her hip movements in her open robe, putting her pudenda in front of his face. She suddenly stopped and regained her sitting posture. "Your turn."

Roger was trying to practice extreme self-control. He worried that any movement would stimulate him to erection, so he continued with his slow, sexy, and sonorous sentences, telling himself that women are more stimulated by thought and imagination rather than by the sight of men's organs. By the end of his soliloquy, he thought he saw her pupils dilating.

As Jessica stood up, she tossed her robe aside and started a series of poses.

"No fair," cried Roger. "You're doing hot yoga!"

"Exactly, you said anything but touching," as she attained the triangle position, facing him and smiling all the while.

"Your two minutes are up," Roger noted.

"But I can stay this way much longer. I'm not doing a thing. You never said we had to stay seated."

Roger was having difficulty constructing sentences. He was also aware that her actions were producing a strong physiologic response, which she could see. Her steady posture, legs spread apart without a quiver, indicated her strength and self-control.

"One minute left in your turn, Roger."

"If I concede the game, can we go to bed?" he asked.

"Aw, I was just getting started," as she worked her pelvic muscles to twitch her labia.

Roger leapt to his feet, snatched her around the waist, and carried her to the bedroom. "I call this a flying fuck forfeit," she laughed.

CHAPTER 21

"Well, Boss, how was the weekend? With all that rain, I bet you didn't get in much skiing," Marsha said when she entered the office.

"No skiing, but I had a great weekend, thank you. I see an email from Steiner. He's ready to discuss my draft budget. Set up an appointment time, please. And leave Thursday open after 3 p.m. for my lesson."

"Your lesson? Learning to fly? Learning Russian? Piano?"

"No, fly fishing. Jessica is going to start teaching me." Marsha's arched eyebrows provided her only answer.

Roger said, "I'd like you to start making the arrangements for the California trip next month. I've committed to speaking at both UC Berkeley and UCSF and need two days at each place to interview those two candidates I told you about. Book me into San Francisco Four Seasons for the whole time. I can take BART over to Berkeley. San Francisco is a lot more interesting than Berkeley."

"I'll get started on it this morning. At 9, Anna Jimenez from Human Resources is coming by for a few minutes. Something about incomplete paperwork."

Anna Jiminez quickly explained the reason for the visit. "When you filled out your employment forms, you didn't complete the question on race. Given your background, that may be a sensitive topic, so I didn't fill in the blank for you," she said as she placed the form in front of him.

Roger remembered leaving the question unanswered. "Why is it important?"

"Stupid bureaucracy. The federal government is always asking about race to measure if we are hiring enough minorities. I'm sorry to bother you."

He looked at the boxes: White, Black, Indigenous American, Latin, Asian, or Other? He was silly to let a simple question give him sudden heartburn. With his pen, he paused over the White box, then stroked the last box, Other. What was his race? Maybe his genetic analysis would help him answer that question.

Anna Jiminez was leaving when Marsha approached. "The protesters are back. This time they brought a drum." She handed him a copy of the day's student newspaper. The headline read; *Professor gets made-to-measure body.* Under that were two pictures of Roger—his hospital photo of two years earlier and another from the press announcement of his appointment. A lengthy article described his transplant surgery, including the donor selection process and preparation. A third picture showed Harbin's prison-like structure, colloquially known there as The Farm. A Chinese student journalist in Shan's class had authored the piece with assistance from a cousin in Harbin. The student journalist had done his work, including researching the scientific literature in both English and Chinese.

Roger felt a tinge of nausea, followed by a flush of anger. He called Stan Hamilton to ask, "What the hell is going on? Have you seen this morning's student newspaper?"

"I'm reading it right now. I'll try to reach Professor Shan. In the meantime, I suggest you leave the campus and be unavailable to any media until we can sort this out. I'll call you in a few hours. Buy a cheap phone with a different number. Your assistant can distribute the number to a select few people. Avoid anyone that looks like press or television."

"I'll take your advice. Please call me as soon as you have anything new."

The moment he regained the privacy of his office, Roger called Jessica on her private number. "I can't discuss it now, but can I see you sometime today? Lunch, dinner, or whatever. I need your help with a problem."

"Of course, Roger. You sound very concerned. Are you sick or something?"

"No, it's a personal problem. You're one of the few people I can talk to about it."

"I'm jammed until about 5. What about an early dinner at my apartment? We can do take-out from there. Would 5:30 be okay?"

"Thanks, Jessica. I'll see you then."

Thirty minutes of useless attempts to deal with his Institute business convinced Roger that he had to clear his mind. When Marsha returned from buying him a cheap cell phone, he said, "I'm not feeling great. I'm going home for the afternoon. Don't bother me unless Dr. Hamilton is looking for me. I'll be alright tomorrow."

"Take care of yourself, boss. I'll watch things here."

Back at his apartment, Roger was pleased to see the seventy-foot salt-water lap pool was not in use. He took the opportunity to change into his trunks and plunge into a full hour of non-stop crawl stroke, counting each turn to himself. The exercise had its desired effect. The anger and frustration of the morning events melted away to composure and determination. He emerged tired enough for a thirty-minute nap. When he checked his telephone, he saw several numbers he did not recognize. He assumed the media was chasing him. He placed his medications and shaving gear into his backpack.

Jessica's television was playing the local news when he arrived. They hugged and kissed. "I took the liberty of preparing a shaker of your favorite Manhattans. Now or later?" she asked.

"Not now, but soon. Let me tell you what happened this morning." Roger handed her the student newspaper and recounted the day's events, adding, "They portray me as a villain for accepting a transplant in China. It's not like I went there to buy a kidney or a liver like hundreds of Americans do every year. And the university is being blamed for rewarding me. It's unfair."

"That's terrible. You've spoken out against capital punishment. You've never supported the Chinese policies. You're innocent, but you'll have to defend yourself. How can I help?"

"I don't know, but when this happened, you were the first person I wanted to contact. I'm sorry to burden you with this," Roger replied.

"Come on, that's what a friend is for. I'll help you any way I can. Is the University threatening to fire you or anything like that?"

"No mention of that, but I could become the sacrificial lamb if they needed one."

Jessica asked, "Does Peter Weaver know of this?"

"Hamilton didn't mention it."

"I think we should let Peter know. I'll text him and ask him to call us."

As they talked, the news channel showed the demonstrators in front of Roger's office and then interviewed the author of the newspaper article. The segment created the impression that Roger was an extreme example of Americans traveling to China for organ transplants.

"This is unfair. You need a lawyer," Jessica advised.

"Why? I didn't do anything wrong."

"But you are being damaged as they trash your reputation. Your job and career are in danger. You have to protect yourself."

"You're a lawyer. Could you help me?"

"I can't be your lawyer. Do you have a lawyer that you know?"

Roger was frowning. "Not really. Can you suggest someone?"

"I'll make a few calls and get you some help." She took her phone into her bedroom and closed the door while Roger re-read the student article until Jessica returned.

Jessica explained, "Okay, here's what I did. I called a good friend at the ACLU. She pointed out that they were more likely to be protecting the students' second amendment rights. My dad suggested Phillip Cohen, who I've known all my life. He's Uncle Phil to me. When I called him, he said he'd be glad to help. He suggests meeting at his office tomorrow morning at 9."

"Thanks for your help. I wouldn't have thought of a lawyer. Can you come with me?"

"I'll go to introduce you, but I won't stay for your meeting. I'm going to call for food delivery. What do you feel like? Italian? Thai? American?"

"Anything but Chinese. Surprise me."

As they waited, Roger's new phone sounded Dr. Hamilton's call. "Dr. Scully, let me bring you up to date. Professor Shan denies any responsibility for either the article or the new demonstration. The President and I think this story will die in a few days if we don't over-react. I suggest you not come onto campus or give interviews to the media. Of course, it's up to you."

"I understand. I may leave town for a few days."

"Good idea. We've set up a meeting with Shan and some others on Tuesday afternoon. I'd like you to attend."

"Of course, I'll come, but I may bring my attorney if you don't mind."

"I'm surprised, but I can understand why. Bring your attorney at 3 in the afternoon. We're not giving out the location at the moment because we don't trust Shan and his protesters. I'll be in touch on Tuesday morning."

"Thank you. I look forward to your call."

Jessica was watching and listening attentively. "I'm glad you'll have an attorney. How do you intend to stay hidden?"

"First, can I stay here overnight? I wouldn't be surprised at the media staking out my apartment."

"Of course. Stay as long as you need to."

"I'd like to fly to Boston and see my folks for the weekend. Wanna come? I need to escape, and you can meet my folks."

"Thanks for the invite, but you're rushing it a little, meeting parents. I've also got a full schedule for my dad. When are you leaving?" asked Jessica.

"Tomorrow afternoon. I'll book a flight right now. I'll be back Monday."

"Make sure you wear a mask. I worry about you flying during the epidemic."

"Don't worry. I'll be careful."

Jessica drove them to Phillip Cohen's office. The receptionist recognized Jessica with a bright smile and escorted them into the attorney's office. Jessica rushed to Cohen with a warm hug, after which she introduced Roger. "I'm leaving immediately. I don't want to screw up attorney-client privilege." She waved her hand and left.

Cohen gestured to a young woman dressed in a straight skirt, black sweater, and tailored blazer. "Dr. Scully, let me introduce Susan Sachs, my associate. She'll do any research. Have a seat at the table and tell me your story."

Roger spent twenty minutes reciting the story from the accident in Tibet, through Chengdu and Harbin, to his present position and the protesters. Cohen interrupted only once when Roger displayed the photo of his naked torso immediately after the hemicorporectomy. "Would you mind sending that to Susan? It might be a useful exhibit."

At the end of the recitation, Cohen addressed Roger. "We can help you. I'll go with you to that meeting on Tuesday. I'll turn you over to Susan for a while to get more information concerning your background and training. Do you have any questions for me?"

"Yeah, what about paying for your services?"

"I bill at $700 per hour, Susan at $300. If we use our paralegals, they cost $100 per hour. Susan will introduce you to our billing office on the way out."

CHAPTER 22

While waiting for the Boston flight, he called Marsha, whom he had texted about his weekend plans. "Those people are still shuffling around in front of our building. I've told all callers you are out of town. Check your email. The University just put out a notice about the virus."

The University email was ominous, announcing that everyone on campus should wear masks. They stressed that everyone should avoid all unnecessary gatherings. New policies about classes would follow shortly. Everyone should read the CDC guidelines on the web. Roger wore his mask throughout the trip, tried to avoid proximity to other passengers, and studied the internet for the latest developments. Epidemiologists were unanimous in their dire predictions.

Roger appeared at his parents' restaurant for the first time since the transplant. The maître d', who had known him since his teen years, gave him a big hug and welcomed him back as though Roger had not changed. They were half an hour from the regular opening time. Mr. Scully spoke up, "Frank, let's get dinner started early. We've got tickets for the Bruins game tonight."

Roger was pleasantly surprised. Tickets for a semifinal against the Rangers were scarce.

"Dad, those must have cost a fortune."

"Don't worry, Rog. Someone owed me a favor."

At the rink, Roger excused himself during warmups. He soon resumed his seat and handed his father a beer.

"Rog, if you got away from those academic crazies, you could work here, and we could have season tickets for both the Sox and the Bruins."

"I'm only dealing with one guy you consider crazy. He has a legitimate cause concerning the Chinese. It's my bad luck that I ended up in the center of the issue. We have a meeting early next week when I hope to settle the whole affair."

"He still sounds like an asshole. Don't let him push you around."

"Let's enjoy the game. I haven't seen the Rangers play here for years."

Back in his Natick bedroom, Roger called Jessica. "Has the publicity calmed down there?"

"Nothing about you on the news today. I drove by your office this afternoon and saw no signs and no protests. Maybe this will all blow over. People are more concerned about the virus than human rights in China."

"I hope so, but I'm not confident. Can we have dinner Monday night?"

"Love to, and you can stay at my place again. It's a good idea to keep a low profile, at least until you have your Tuesday meeting with that creepy professor. Did you see your CNN coverage last night?"

"Yeah, I watched it with my folks. Mom was in tears. Dad wants to fly to Denver and punch out that guy's lights. I couldn't find anything in the Globe today, which made me happy. They didn't pick up on the Denver story as having a Boston connection. On Monday,

I have a late afternoon appointment at the University. What time should I appear at your place?"

"I'll leave early and be there at 5," Jessica answered.

"Thank you for being so supportive."

On the return flight, Roger worried more about his genetic analysis results than Professor Shan's cause. He had done nothing wrong in accepting the transplant. It was unfair for Shan to make an example of him. The four-and-a-half-hour flight felt like a full day. When he landed, he found an email from Marsha, notifying him that he had an appointment Tuesday afternoon with Dr. Gillespie in Genetics. He felt his stomach rise when he read the message.

Jessica greeted him with a long embrace and a wide smile. "Welcome back, my stud. I missed you."

"And I missed you. I would like you to meet my parents soon. I've decided I'm in love with you."

"I feel something, too, but we've only known each other a month. Let's enjoy each other and see what happens."

"Suits me," said Roger. "I'm on a time change, so I'm hungry. What are our dinner plans?"

"I made lasagna and salad, so it's my cooking tonight. Cocktails are made and in the fridge. Want yours now?"

"Absolutely, as soon as I wash up."

Over drinks and dinner, Roger recounted his weekend in Boston. His pleasure with the weekend with his parents was apparent. Jessica commented, "It sounds like the Boston weekend was a good idea. Any new thoughts on your meeting tomorrow with that Shan guy?"

"Nothing new. My dad wants to punch him out. We'll see what the University says at the meeting."

"I'm confident you have a great lawyer. Just listen to anything he tells you. Did you wear a mask all the time on your trip?"

"Yeah, but I was surprised to see so few others covered up. Even the flight attendants were not wearing any masks. I have a pretty good supply. Tomorrow I'll get you a few."

They were in bed by 8 p.m., enjoying each other's bodies. Jessica wiped from Roger's mind any concern about the following morning.

He was at his office an hour before his scheduled meeting. Marsha, wearing a mask, updated him on administrative issues and reminded him of his late afternoon appointment with Dr. Gillespie. He felt his stomach roll. He now had something other than demonstrators and viruses to consider.

The meeting with Shan in Hamilton's office was brief. All attendees wore masks. Shan opened the discussion by saying, "I apologize for the demonstrators last week. Those were a few over-enthusiastic students acting without supervision. They stopped demonstrating when I explained we were planning a meeting to negotiate the issue."

Vice President Hamilton nodded and asked, "What do you want the University to do?"

"Our group thinks it was wrong to hire Professor Scully. China has a well-known medical tourism industry based on selling organs. By hiring Professor Scully, you promote China's terrible program. You should dismiss him," Shan answered.

Roger felt his anger welling up and his face getting red. Trying to maintain his composure, and with Phil Cohen looking aghast, Roger shoved a photo across the table. Facing Shan, he said, "Here's a picture of me a little more than a year ago. No lower torso, no legs, no future. I was about to kill myself. Chinese doctors saved my life. What would you have done? Become a dependent cripple for life?"

"Did you ask where they got the donor?"

"They explained to me that donors were persons already condemned to death for criminal convictions. The donors elect death under anesthesia instead of being shot."

"It's not right that they killed a man to make his body available to you."

"He had already been sentenced to death. They were going to kill him anyway. My needs had nothing to do with their decision. The prisoner and his family consented to donate his body."

"Do you approve of the treatment of the Uyghurs? Do you approve of the extent of capital punishment in China?"

"You don't know the whole story. Look at me. I resemble a Uyghur, and I suffered for it in China. I have publicly spoken out against capital punishment. So you want the University to fire me for something you consider a misdeed? Does that help anyone?"

Hamilton spoke up. "The best solution may be to do nothing. Why keep this story alive? The University is not going to fire Professor Scully. Two wrongs do not make a right. Professor Shan, if your students wish to continue protesting against Chinese practices, that is their privilege. It is not their right to try to ruin the career of an innocent man."

Shan leaned down and said, "I'm sorry. I have no animus toward Professor Scully. I did not know the circumstances. I withdraw my request for his dismissal. Professor Scully, I apologize to you. I would shake your hand if it weren't against the new regulations."

In less than sixty minutes, Roger Scully had won his first battle in academic politics.

He arrived in Brenda Gillespie's office, looking drawn and tired from the previous meeting. He forced a smile at her greeting. "What can you tell me about my genes?"

"Your lab work is most unusual. As you remember, we did these analyses because of your concern that, as a chimera, your DNA typing might show characteristics of both DNA sources. Well, you were correct. The majority of specimens showed a DNA pattern quite different from your blood specimen, which we assume is your original Scully pattern. Buccal swabs showed only a small portion of samples with the Scully gene. Your sperm showed both DNA patterns, with Scully genes appearing in about one-third of the spermatozoa examined."

"So I might father a child with my original DNA type?"

"That's a distinct possibility."

"Could I do in-vitro fertilization and select the right sperm?"

"My lab won't help you. It's unethical to mess with sperm for that kind of thing. Not saying you won't be able to find another lab to help you."

"I'll have to think about it in the future. I'm excited that Scully sperm still exist in my body. Thank you for doing all of this."

"Do you have any problem if we write this up for publication? We would never identify you."

Roger replied, "Provided you don't mention either the nature of the transplant or the racial differences. Either of those facts would immediately identify me."

"I'll show you the paper before I submit it. You can refuse permission to publish."

"That sounds fair. I've got the answers I wanted, and I'm tired from my flight today. Thank you again. I'm on my way."

Roger was anxious to share his news with Jessica. He had suddenly lost some of his fatigue. Waiting in a traffic jam, he wondered why he wanted to tell Jessica. They had never discussed marriage, let alone children. Would a discussion of his sperm disturb her? Despite these reservations, he still wanted to share the news.

Jessica greeted him with a huge hug and several deep kisses. "Welcome back, my darling man. I'm so glad to get you back. Anything new?"

"Shan backed down, and the University supported me. That issue is finished. I have some more exciting and positive news." Roger was beaming.

"So, tell me!"

"A few weeks ago, I had a lot of DNA testing done. You had enough biology to know that DNA decides everything in your body. This afternoon, I found out that some of my sperm have the original Roger Scully DNA and not just donor DNA."

Jessica looked puzzled. "And?"

"It means I am capable of fathering a Caucasian child related to the original me, Roger."

"I'm not sure I understand. Why is that important?"

"Well, I might have a white son or daughter!" Roger replied with enthusiasm.

"It sounds like you would prefer a white child instead of an Asian. Isn't that a bit racist?"

Roger frowned, "You don't understand."

"You're right. I don't understand. For me, it doesn't matter about the skin color of the Roger Scully that I adore. I'm a bit shocked that you would discriminate against Asians when you are one. Think about what you imply."

Roger sat and put his face in his hands. "Oh, shit. I'm confused. Who am I? I don't want to be a racist. The Chinese saved my life and were wonderful to me."

"Oh, ease up, Roger. You had good news today, getting rid of that protest thing. Stop worrying about your skin color. I'm more worried about this virus epidemic. You're a doctor. What should we be doing about the virus?"

CHAPTER 23

Roger responded to Jessica's question. "This virus is very scary. Epidemiology is not my specialty. Tomorrow I'll call Jack Palmer, the epidemiologist, over in Preventive Medicine. Two years ago, he was interested in analyzing ER admissions. I must be at high risk because I am immunocompromised by being on cyclosporine. I don't dare any virus exposure."

By 8 the next morning, Roger and Marsha were in the University office. He was trying to plan a strategy for dealing with the virus. "Cancel my California trip. I'm doing no travel for the next few months. I'm going to work from home and not come to the office. I'm at high risk for the virus. You won't see me for a while. Put the budget figures on a flash drive for me to take home."

He called Jack Palmer. "Jack, it's Roger Scully. Do you remember me from our discussions in the ER a few years ago?"

"Yeah, of course. I understand you're quite a celebrity now. How's it going?"

"I need your opinion about Covid. I'm immunocompromised from my transplant. What should I do?"

Palmer replied, "Stay away from people as much as you can. Always wear a mask if you are around others, and wash your hands. You know the drill. You might find a cave and become a hermit for the next year or so."

"Year or so?"

"Oh yes, we're going to have this virus for at least a year. Epidemiologists have predicted this for decades. I've had three months of freeze-dried food for the past twenty years because the food supply might break down."

"You're kidding!"

"I'm serious. In your spare time, read a book called *The Great Influenza* that describes what might happen if we have a pandemic like the flu of 1918. Almost no one except the epidemiologists and infectious disease docs are taking this seriously enough. Hole up somewhere and don't see people."

"I'll take your advice, Jack. Thank you. And stay well yourself."

As he prepared to leave the office, his screen lit up with a long message from the University President. The University was shutting down many of its operations. Roger felt a sudden sense of urgency. His brain shifted into the gear he had used in his years of dealing with multiple serious casualties. He called Jessica, and after explaining the University's actions and Jack Palmer's advice, said, in his calm, slow, and serious voice, "I'm going to leave town. I need to get three months of my prescriptions and a supply of food and leave for the mountains, away from people."

"Where are you going to go?"

"I might go to Loveland and rent a cabin there."

"You're welcome to use my place." Jessica offered.

"That's very kind, but what about you?"

"I might join you. Everything is in turmoil here, and after today,

I'll be working from home. Can I see you at my place in a few hours?"

"Good idea. I'm going to get my prescriptions, some food, and a lot of cash. Will you be home by 2?"

"Come at 1, and we can have lunch while we plan this out."

"See you then. And wear your mask at the office!"

After a short discussion with Marsha, he picked up ten respirator masks from the hospital; they were already limiting the number issued. He headed to Arvada, his Denver's source for freeze-dried food. He knew it well from when he and Joanne would backpack into the hills. At his bank, he caused a stir when he handed the teller a check for $10,000, "In twenties, please." The pharmacist understood his need for three months of cyclosporine but pointed out that only two months of capsules were in stock. Roger accepted those, realizing he could order more at the pharmacy in Loveland. By noon he was loading his camping gear into the Jeep.

Jessica had lunch prepared when he arrived. He explained his morning's actions.

"Wow, you move fast. You must be the best-organized man I know."

"It's the personality of an ER doc. You never know what's coming through those doors and how many of them. You learn to organize and prioritize. Let's discuss our plan. This virus pandemic is long-term. It won't disappear in a week or a month. Any vaccine won't be ready until next year, at the earliest."

"What about treatment?" Jessica asked with a concerned look.

"We don't have one yet. The pharmaceutical industry has a poor record in discovering anti-virals, so we don't expect new treatments in the next six months. My immune system is not going to improve. That means I have to isolate to some degree for the next six to twelve months, minimum."

"That long? I didn't think of anything that far out."

"I'm afraid I'm correct. I appreciate the loan of your cabin. I hope you'll join me there. At least we can take walks and hikes, and even go camping. If we live together, you've got to agree to kick me out at any time. I can find another place. We're both optimistic but haven't tried living together, which is always uncertain until you've done it. We have to be honest with each other at all times."

Jessica nodded, "I understand you. Let's give it a try. I guarantee I'll have no problem kicking you out if it's not working. Let's do some planning. Internet service is good at the cabin. We should both be able to work from there. I have a folding table we can use as a second desk. What about food?" Jessica asked.

"I loaded the Jeep with about three months of freeze-dried food for emergencies, such as food deliveries stopping. Let's make one major shopping list for essentials like canned goods, pasta, etcetera. You know what you have at the cabin now, but we should be independent for at least three months. Trader Joe's has some excellent packaged products with infinite shelf life. We should also think about planting a vegetable garden."

Jessica was shaking her head. "Vegetable garden? You do think long-term. I like that idea. The cabin pantry has a good supply of canned food and some beans and dried things. Remember that I'm from Mormon stock; we prepare for uncertainty."

"I'll stop for wine, beer, and booze. I suggest you do the grocery shopping, wearing a mask. I want to leave this afternoon. When can you join me?"

"I'll be there late tomorrow. I'm having dinner with my folks tonight. They'll be surprised at our plans, but they'll understand. What about your job?"

"The University canceled all the usual meetings. I told Marsha my plans, and she'll work from home after tomorrow. She'll cancel the California trip. Everything is on indefinite hold. I don't know how I'm supposed to recruit faculty and build an institute when everything is shut down."

"You make it sound much worse than the President or his advisors," Jessica said.

"Listen to the epidemiologists. They're the smart ones. The world is in a mess for at least a year, maybe more. Today, we concentrate on planning our survival for the next six months, but the bigger challenge is our future together."

"I'm canceling my tomorrow meetings. I'll spend the morning organizing things so I can work remotely. I should be at Loveland by 6 or 7. Shall we do the Bistro?" Jessica asked.

"No, lovely lady. You have to understand the need to isolate. Bars and restaurants are off-limits for us. Your dad can close them or leave them open, but we're not going to them."

"Okay. I'll pick up dinner at Trader Joes on the way. You should be able to find something tonight in the chest freezer if there's nothing in the fridge."

After lunch, he stopped at his favorite liquor store as he prepared to depart Denver for Loveland. He was surprised to find the store more crowded than usual. None of the staff and only one other customer were wearing masks. He overheard another customer say to his wife, "That Chinese guy is probably the one who brought the virus to Denver." Roger inwardly flinched but ignored the comment. His wine and liquor order filled two boxes. A quick stop at Home Depot supplied him with several packets of vegetable seeds. At his last Denver stop, the post office, he completed a change of address form with Loveland as his new address. On arrival at Loveland, he filled his gas tank.

The security guard at the gated development checked his tablet; Roger Scully was clear to enter. Jessica's key opened the garage, so he unloaded the Jeep inside. He sent a text to Jessica announcing his arrival, then called his father to report his move.

His father answered, "I'm glad you called. Today the Governor ordered us to shut the restaurant because of this virus thing. I was about to call you to ask your opinion. No one seems to know how long the lockdown will last. Do I fire the staff, put them on vacation, or what?"

Roger replied, "Listen to Fauci and the epidemiologists. We're in trouble for months, at a minimum. It could be years. I have no idea what kinds of relief you might get from the city, state, or federal governments. Right now, they all seem confused. I don't know much more than you. I checked the CDC website, and it's not helpful. I plan on staying here at least three months before I head back to the city."

"We may have to close the restaurant. I can't afford rent with no income. We might decide to retire."

"That might be a good idea. In the meantime, wear a mask, avoid everyone, and wash your hands often, like you always taught me. Call me anytime, but remember the time difference."

As Roger ate his reheated frozen chili, Covid dominated every television news broadcast. The President, urging calm, disagreed with every infectious disease expert or epidemiologist. The stock market was crashing. Roger felt reassured by his decision to flee Denver.

When Jessica called, he could hear the tension in her voice. "It's a madhouse here. Dad is in non-stop meetings with public health officials, the restaurant association, and God knows who else. I can't help him, and I can't get anything done here. I should be there tomorrow by 3 or 4 o'clock."

"Wear your mask and stay away from everyone. Shop early before there are any crowds. And fill your gas tank when you get to Loveland."

"Why the gas?" Jessica asked.

"If the epidemic is as big as in 1918, there may be no trucks hauling gas."

"If you say so. I'll be glad to see you in Loveland."

The next day, Roger spent most of his time organizing an inventory of food and drink. He also strolled the property, considering its potential for a vegetable garden. A series of emails indicated that his medical colleagues were organizing call rosters for the ER and acute care units. Roger had a short pang of guilt, but his immunocompromised state made him unsuitable for any patient care. He would have to sit this one out.

CHAPTER 24

Jessica said, "I have enough work to keep me busy for the next week or more, but then what? What are we going to do with all this time?"

"There's almost nothing I can do for the University right now. I need to catch up with my science reading, so the internet is a godsend. We can do some hiking and camping. If we're alone, that's very safe. And I'm going to write a book!"

"A book? What about?"

"My life. I even have a title. *Chimera Conflict* will deal with the issues I've felt since my transplant. Every year we now have thousands of new chimeras created through transplants. My experience may help some of them understand the complications and conflicts they might endure."

As he arranged himself at the computer, Jessica said, "I've never seen you so enthused about anything other than sex!"

"Well, I am enthused. I want to write my biography. It might be inspiring to others. You've seen the picture of me in Chengdu. Look at all the positive things that have happened to me since. And you're one of those positive things. Since I'm forced into a paid vacation, it's a perfect way to spend some time."

"Go to it. I'm going to inventory the freezer and deal with emails from my dad."

As he opened his laptop, he noticed an email from Lushan. With a dry mouth he read:

DearZichang

I hope this finds you well and free of the terrible virus. So far, I have escaped infection but spend most of my waking hours in protective gear at the hospital. We are very busy trying to save so many people.

I am writing to tell you I am now five months pregnant. You didn't notice my body changes before you left. When it became clear that we would separate, I had my IUD removed in the hope that I could be left with your baby as a remembrance. My plan succeeded and your son is due to arrive about September 1. I take full responsibility for this pregnancy. I will not expect any support, money or otherwise, from you. My new job has excellent on-site childcare so I will be able to take him to work and see him through the day. I start there June 15. I had several offers but this one attracted me most because of the nursery facilities.

When we discussed the possibility of parenting, I told you I wanted my children to benefit from Chinese culture and education. I have not changed my mind so please do not try to persuade me to move to America. I still love you and hope you find a proper American wife to have those children we talked about. Please keep me informed about your life and career.

Love, Lushan

Roger read the letter three times before he printed it. From the printer he walked to the counter they used as a bar. He was pouring a two-ounce shot of Jim Beam when Jessica walked in.

"Whoa, Roger. Ten in the morning's a little early for that," she said. "Are you okay, you look like something is wrong."

Handing her the printout, Roger said, "We need to talk."

"Wait a moment. I want to re-read it." When she finished, she asked, "How do you feel about this?"

"It's not fair. Wendy should have discussed this before. Now I'll have a son I can't relate to. I'm pissed at her getting pregnant without telling me her plans."

"Roger, it seems that Lushan is a very intelligent woman with her view of her future. She planned the pregnancy and now seems to be well-organized for career and childcare. She's not asking you for anything, so you have no responsibility. I admire her," Jessica said with a faint smile.

"I will want to see my son," Roger said. His lips quivered and Jessica noticed a tear rolling down his left cheek.

"You have lots of time to think about that. Until further notice, travel to China is impossible and it may be years before you can visit."

"You don't understand. If Joanne had lived, she would probably be pregnant right now, or maybe even delivered. We had plans," Roger said.

"I understand that; you told me the story. But you have to realize that the future is what counts. If we stay together, we can have our child in a few years. Let's make this relationship work and look ahead, not back," she said as she stroked his back.

Jessica's phone interrupted them. Roger only heard her responses. "Yes, Alan, I'm at my cottage with Roger. We're both fine. Are you okay?"—pause—"No, you can't come visit. Roger has health issues so he's at high risk. We are seeing nobody for the near future."—pause—"I'm sorry to disappoint you, Alan, but that's the way it has to be. Are you at your cabin here in Loveland?"—pause—"You see, that makes it even more important that you not visit right now. You're living with three other guys and who knows what their exposure is. I'd love to see you but this is just not the time. Let's keep in touch until things are clearer. OK?"—pause—"Thank you for understanding. Stay healthy and call often, Bye for now."

Jessica turned to Roger. "That was Alan, your ski instructor. He's living here in Loveland and wanted to visit. I think you heard me tell him that there is no visiting. Did I do the right thing?"

Roger nodded, "Yeah, certainly but you're giving up your friends to protect me. I appreciate what you're doing but I'm not sure I'm worth it."

"Don't spout nonsense. Finish that drink, put on a jacket and your hiking boots. We're going for a long walk to check the snow level on the mountain. I don't need a mask, do I?"

"No, but keep one in your pocket in case we meet anyone on the trail."

They said little on their ninety-minute hike. Roger had his camera to capture some spring foliage against the clear Colorado sky. He commented, "You had a good idea," as he removed his hiking boots. "I feel better already."

Over left-over lasagna and Chianti, they discussed Roger's proposed garden plans, including a small greenhouse he had discovered on Amazon. He could get an early start on his vegetables. Jessica expressed concern over her career. She could not fathom starting as a junior associate working from the cabin. The word *virtual* was beginning to appear and applied to meetings, lectures, and even weddings. Jessica announced that she could not envision a virtual career in a mountain cabin with no colleagues, no law books, and no clients. "Screw it. I'll become a cook or gardener or photographer for the next six months or a year," she announced.

"All positive ideas. And you can teach me to fly cast," he smiled.

"I have a better idea. Let's shower together and see what happens," she said.

CHAPTER 25

Jessica and Roger soon settled into a comfortable routine. Roger made breakfast, then headed for his laptop to search medical literature, answer emails, and write the first few chapters of his new novel, *Chimera Conflict*. Jessica responded to emails, including correspondence with two Boulder law firms interested in hiring her. They took a ten o'clock coffee break on the back patio, weather permitting, often discussing the proposed garden layout. Jessica prepared a light lunch which they often took on a nearby almost-deserted trail. About a mile into the forest, a warped grey picnic table waited patiently. On returning, they shared a pot of tea before Roger returned to his writing while Jessica prepared dinner. Much of their conversation centered around Jessica's career. She contacted the Sierra Club and a few other not-for-profit organizations, favoring that type of activity over the usual business of law firms.

A month after their move to the cabin, Jessica observed over after-dinner coffee, "You know, we act like an old married couple."

"So let's do it. Will you marry me? A month or so ago, you said I was rushing it when I suggested you meet my folks. I feel even stronger now about us. I love you and want to spend the rest of my life with you."

Jessica replied, "Since I met you, I've always worried about competing with Joanne, who is so important to your history. I was less worried about Wendy, although her email about the pregnancy gave me a start."

"You're not competing with either of them. The past is over. I want to look forward. Your idea of working in the environmental section would make raising children easier than being in a high-powered law firm. I think we would be good parents. You've said you want children." Roger said.

"I'll say yes if you carry me into the bedroom," she smiled.

Roger stood up, reached over her sitting on the couch, and swept her over his right shoulder. To sounds of her laughter, he said, "You're always testing my strength. I haven't carried you since we played the Shibumi game."

Lying quietly after an hour of vigorous passion, they discussed marriage arrangements. Jessica observed, "You know, there's an advantage to this Covid problem. Normally, it's a big deal if the governor's daughter marries. Today, people are just not doing events that bring all the family and friends. I need to discuss it with my folks, but I suggest we elope here to Loveland and have the celebration after the epidemic."

"Great idea. My folks will feel a little left out, but they can't travel now. We can celebrate when the epidemic is over."

For breakfast the next morning, Roger duplicated an earlier one: mushroom omelet with Mimosas. Jessica glowed with pleasure after affecting her surprise at the meal.

Jessica asked, "Does elopement mean we don't get any honeymoon?"

Roger smiled, "I've given that some thought already. I remember you were interested in the Tibet trek to photograph a snow leopard. Let's take the trip I never completed."

"What a great idea!

"I was hoping we might get to this conversation, so I brought my old Tibet file from home," Roger said. "Read it but also check out visa requirements. I have no idea what the Chinese want now for information."

Immediately after breakfast, with some trepidation, Jessica called Denver. "Good morning, Mom. I have a surprise for you."

"Oh, hi dear. I hadn't heard from you the past few days. How's it going?" her mother asked.

"Great, we're going to get married. Soon, here in Loveland."

"What? I haven't even met your Roger. Why so sudden? Are you pregnant?"

Jessica was envisioning her mother's face. "No, Mom. We love each other so much, and the pandemic has fouled up everything normal. People are eloping all over because of the restrictions. I know you always thought I would have a big wedding in Denver, but it's impossible. If you and Dad bring up Bishop Smith, he can do the ceremony right here. When the pandemic ends, you can throw us a big reception at the mansion."

Her mother was calm. "I'm not going to argue with you. You always know what you're doing. Dad was impressed with Roger, so I'm not questioning your choice. When do you want to do this?"

Jessica had anticipated the question. "As soon as possible, even his week. If we wait, more and more people will hear about it, and a mob will show up even without an invitation. I want Norma and Marlene as witnesses; they're living here in Loveland. You and Dad are the only guests. Roger's folks are in Boston and can't travel."

"You sound determined. Dad is home this morning, so we'll discuss it, and I'll call you back. Is everything else okay? You're both well?"

"Yes, we're both great. Thank you for understanding. Some mothers would have thrown a fit," Jessica said.

"I never throw fits. I'll call you later this morning."

When Roger called his parents to explain their plans, they were happy for him but disappointed they could not attend. His mother asked, "What are you doing about rings?"

"Ohmygod, I haven't even thought about it. I can't go shopping," Roger said.

His mother had a suggestion. "Why don't I Fedex my mother's wedding ring. I was always hoping you might use it when you found someone to replace Joanne. Will you take it?"

"I know the ring. That's a beautiful suggestion. Thank you for solving my problem. I can't wait for you to meet Jessica; I sure you will approve."

"I know you've chosen well. I'm starting to cry, so I'll give the phone to Dad."

Over the next few minutes, the two men discussed the still-forming wedding plans, the final closure of the restaurant, and news about a few friends and family. Roger left the conversation happy, and immediately shared the news with Jessica.

CHAPTER 26

As he gathered his thoughts for the novel, the doorbell rang. It was two days since his conversation with his parents; Roger expected a Fedex. Instead, a postal employee handed him a registered letter to accept with a signature at the front door. The return address said Colorado State Board of Medical Examiners.

What's this? I'm not due for re-licensing yet?

The letter read:

The Board hereby notifies you of a complaint lodged against you concerning your practice of medicine in the State of Colorado. It is alleged that you are not Roger E. Scully, as you claim, but are impersonating him. Impersonation of a medical person is a felony in this state. To investigate this matter, we suggest an informal hearing with the Board, following which the Board will decide upon the further pursuit of this matter. You are entitled to be represented by counsel at the hearing. In the meantime, you are not to practice medicine. Your prescribing privileges are now suspended.

Enclosed with this letter, you will find a copy of the Chinese death certificate of Roger E. Scully, whose name you are now using. You note he was a U.S. citizen who died on January 6, 2019. Cause of death was massive traumatic injuries. Due to the Covid emergency, the hearing will be held virtually at a time convenient to all parties. I suggest you or your attorney call me to schedule the hearing. I look forward to hearing from you shortly.

Yours sincerely,

Edward J. Fellows, MD

Secretary, Colorado State Board of Medical Examiners

He re-read the letter twice. On the death certificate, he recognized the signature of Dengwei Wong.

"Holy shit, Jessica. Look at this," he said, handing her the letter.

Face set in a frown, she read the letter slowly. "This is bad. You need a lawyer, fast," Jessica advised.

"Don't you see? This makes me officially dead," he blurted. "Wong never told me he did that, but I guess when they wheeled my corpse into the morgue, they had to create a death certificate."

Jessica said, "You still have your U.S. passport. That proves you're alive."

"But they issued that passport in the American embassy in China, using my Chinese photo. I wonder how the State Department will view this. Will they revoke my passport?"

"We're going to call Phil Cohen right now. I can probably get through to him," she said as she lifted her cell phone. When Cohen's office referred her to his home, she called there.

"Uncle Phil, it's Jessica. Sorry to bother you, but we have a real crisis. Let Roger explain what's happened."

Roger took the phone and read the Board letter to Cohen, who reacted. "You have a serious problem, as you know. According to the records, you are officially dead. I need to research this, but first, email me the Board letter and the death certificate. Don't reply to the letter until we decide if I'm the right attorney to handle this."

Roger replied, "I'll send it right away."

Cohen continued, "In the meantime, I'll call an old fraternity brother at State and get an informal reading about your passport. Who do you think's behind the Board action? Someone filed that complaint. You must have a serious enemy." Cohen's tone sounded somber.

"I can't think of a single serious enemy. We had the University dust-up over the Uyghur situation, but we resolved the issue. I can't think anyone would be trying to destroy me."

"Someone had to know about the death certificate and went to the trouble to supply the Board with a copy. Think about that. Give me a week to do my research. In the meantime, do nothing about this and don't discuss it with anyone. If the Board or the University contacts you, refer them to me. In the meantime, visit the nearest Social Security office. Take your Social Security card and passport for photo identification. Ask about your account balance to see if they still have you alive."

"Great idea. We'll do that today," Roger said.

He found the closest Social Security office was in Fort Collins, a twenty-minute drive. When he called to ask if they were open, the office informed him that they were functioning for the rest of the day but would close tomorrow because of the virus. Visitors also required masks.

"Let's go, Jessica. We're about to find out if I'm still alive."

At the Social Security office, a uniformed and masked security guard provided Roger with a numbered card and directed them to chairs well away from others in the waiting room. Within twenty minutes, Roger heard his summons to station number three. He obeyed immediately and pushed his passport and Social Security card to the masked woman behind a plastic shield.

"What can I help you with today?" she asked.

"I need to know my balance and find out if the University is making my monthly contributions. She compared his passport photo to his face without touching either document, then wrote his Social Security number on a small pad. "I have to check the computer. Take a seat, and I'll call you. The computer is slow today."

Thirty agonizing minutes later, the clerk recalled Roger. On the slip of paper were his account balance and the date of the last contribution from the University. The clerk did not question his vital status.

When he returned to Jessica, she said, "With your shit-eating grin, I assume you are alive and well."

"Fucking-A. Let's go home and celebrate."

Roger called Phil Cohen as soon as they arrived back at the cabin. Cohen was pleased by the news but had some other thoughts. "When someone dies in a foreign country, that country notifies the country of the deceased's citizenship. There are international agreements for that. However, notifications can take a while. If you die in Switzerland, the U.S. will likely hear the following January when they summarize all deaths. If you die in Russia, it could be years. China is slow and inconsistent, but we can predict notification at some time. In the meantime, we will demand some kind of authentication of that death certificate photo. That gives us more time. Any questions?"

"None. I guess our celebration over Social Security was a bit premature."

"I need you to consider another strategy. If you agree to surrender your medical license at the preliminary hearing voluntarily, the Board will not have to take the action of suspending you. Have you treated any patients since returning to Colorado?"

"No, none at all."

"That's good. It's fair to say you have not been practicing medicine here. If they accept your voluntary withdrawal, the Board can avoid

274

the messy business of suspending you and possibly charging you with a felony. Everybody wins."

"Except me. I lose my license. I'm no longer a doctor," Roger said.

"But you're still a professor with a career while we try to sort out your status. It will be a gutsy move, but one you should consider. You can always apply for relicensing. I'll do some more research on how to protect your identity if and when the Chinese notify the US government of your death"

After the call, Roger and Jessica sat for a while in silence, trying to absorb the situation. Jessica spoke first. "When I first met you, I was charmed and intrigued by your story. At first, it seemed unbelievable. It didn't stop me from falling in love with you, but I had some doubts. The more and better I know you, the more I am convinced by your narrative. I will do anything in my power to support you. There must be a way out of this predicament. How does a person declared dead prove that he is still alive?"

"But who the hell is doing this to me? I don't have any enemies to ruin my life."

"Calm down, Roger. Don't let your anger cloud your reasoning. I see two parts of the problems. One, how do you get your license and your career back? That has to be your priority. Two, who did it, and could they do it again? That is a lesser priority. The lawyers are working on the licensing issue. I see very little that we can do at this time."

"So we just sit around and wait for something to happen?" Roger asked.

"No, we work with the lawyers when they call. If you want to know more about the person that got you into this bind, organize your thoughts. Was this attack from here or abroad?"

Roger bristled, "What do you mean, here or abroad?"

"Well, remember the student demonstrations? At least one of the students had Harbin connections and might still be trying to get rid of you."

"That's true. I hadn't thought of that."

Jessica asked, "Who were the other candidates for your position? I assume there were others."

"I never heard of any, but I suppose it's possible."

"That means you have at least two sources of enemies in this country. Now we should look abroad. Suggestions as to who might want you back in China?"

"Wong once told me he would have me back at any time. I know he needs transplant surgeons. Mr. Moon might want me back in China as an example of outstanding success. If I can't work here, I may have to consider returning to China."

"I can't see you going back there; you still have a job here. How about Lishan turning in that death certificate? She loves you and would be delighted to see you return to China."

He snorted. "She would never do anything like that."

"You don't think so, but don't deceive yourself that you know how a woman thinks," Jessica advised.

"I'd like to kill the son-of-a-bitch that put me into this mess. At this moment, my career is finished. What good is an MD if you can't practice medicine? I want to get my name and career back."

"Of course you do, but the death certificate is a real problem. Doctor Wong has effectively killed off Roger Scully."

"I won't go back to being Wu Zicheng. That's not me."

Jessica shook her head and said, "Shakespeare asked, 'What's in a name?' Maybe you concentrate too much on your Chinese name rather than your identity. You seem to be in conflict with the name and maybe your Uyghur appearance. I think you have a soul, and that soul resides in that great brain of yours."

"I appreciate your confidence, but I still need to reverse that death certificate."

"I have a suggestion. People now post difficult problems on the internet to gather solutions from around the world. Why not try that?" Jessica asked.

"Hey, when I write my memoir, I can then put up a Facebook or other social media page called *Undead Roger Scully*. That will allow the people who read *Chimera Conflict* to contribute a proper ending."

Roger Scully returned to his computer screen displaying the file Chimera Conflict with a smile. Jessica started informing friends and family about their wedding plans she termed 'their Loveland elopement.'

CHAPTER 27

After reading Roger's Tibet file, Jessica turned to the internet to search China visa requirements. "Roger, the website for Chinese visas and Tibet permits makes it looks complicated. They also demand that you appear in person at a consulate; they are developing online application forms."

"Is there a Chinese consulate in Denver?" Roger asked.

"A few months ago, they were planning on opening a consulate. The Chinese have been very active in this area. I know they bought at least one mining property and were in discussions for an engineering company. It's a pattern across the country. They'll own our minerals and our technology," Jessica said. "I'll ask my dad about it when they're here next week."

Jessica was delighted at the heavy gold band wedding ring. "It's beautiful, and it fits! I like the fact that it was your grandmother's. I'll be honored to wear it. My mom insists on bringing us a wedding cake from her favorite bakery. They plan on arriving around noon next Thursday. Bishop Smith will be with them, but they will go back in the evening. Everyone will wear masks except to eat and drink. We can set up the ping-pong table for dinner, so everyone maintains distance.'

"We've plenty of champagne. What should we do about food?" Roger asked.

"Hey, no alcohol. We'll have a Mormon bishop here. I'll call the Bistro. I don't know if they're open for dining, but I'm sure the chef will prepare a takeout dinner for us. Marlene can pick it up on the way here for the ceremony. I'll also ask her to pick up a few bottles of alcohol-free champagne."

"What are we wearing for the ceremony?" Roger asked.

"You will wear a suit and tie."

"And you?" Roger asked.

"Mom is bringing my wedding dress, and I won't let you see it until the ceremony. We have to have some tradition to this."

For the next four days, Jessica ordered food, checked china and cutlery, conferred with her two witnesses, and cleaned every corner of her house. In her spare time, she completed the Chinese visa and Tibet permit forms for both of them. Roger made all dinners and emailed several friends about the forthcoming wedding, promising that there would be a grand party in Denver after the pandemic. They drove into downtown Loveland to obtain a marriage license.

When the black Suburban with the governor's crest on the door pulled into the driveway, Jessica ran, without a mask, to meet her mother. The masked driver opened the rear hatch and carried on high, rather gingerly, a long opaque garment bag. Jessica and her mother directed him into the house.

After the governor introduced the bishop to Roger, the three men sat in Adirondac chairs on the lawn. The bishop explained, "What I'm doing today is unusual, but we live in unusual times. I'd be happier if we had a traditional Mormon ceremony with all parties fully accredited members of the faith. We can't do that, and I'm not advocating Roger go through a year of indoctrination and conversion to our faith. I am licensed to perform the ceremony, but I consider today a civil ceremony rather than a religious one. I would hope that Roger, you will join our faith over the next few years, and then we will have a proper sealing in the temple."

Roger nodded, "Thank you, Bishop, for being so considerate."

Marlene and Norma waved to the men and rushed into the house on arrival.

Thirty minutes later, Norma emerged to announce, "The bride is ready. You three should move to the back patio for the ceremony."

"I thought it was going to be on the lawn," Roger said.

"Women's heels don't work well on a lawn, so we decided on the patio," Norma explained. "Governor, wait in the house so you can escort Jessica."

Roger and Bishop Smith stood at the patio edge, watching the door from the house. Samuel, the governor's regular driver, sat against the wall near the door. Jessica burst through the door on her father's arm, radiant in a traditional white dress with a veil. Roger gulped at her beauty.

The ceremony was brief. Everyone stood, and Samuel took a video with his phone. Ellen Lupen sobbed in silence as she watched her daughter speak her vows.

After the traditional kiss, Roger said to Jessica, "Amazing dress. How did you arrange that?"

"This was Mom's wedding dress. I've been trying it on for years, so I knew it would fit."

"Dinner is served inside," announced Marlene, and they filed to the ping-pong table covered by a pink bedsheet. Norma showed the bishop the label of alcohol-free champagne and filled glasses for everyone. At each place, an individual pizza graced a paper plate. In the center of the table, a traditional three-tiered wedding cake dominated the scene.

Bishop Smith blessed the food, and all present at the table..

Governor Lupen rose from his chair and raised his glass. "To Roger and Jessica Scully, may they have many happy years together."

As Roger was about to reply to the toast, Jessica, remaining seated, said, "Daddy, it's not Doctor and Mrs. Scully. I'm keeping my name."

Roger now spoke with his glass raised. "You've heard the lady. We hadn't discussed the name, but I'm all for it. Now, thank you, Governor and Ellen, for providing me with this wonderful woman I'm proud to call my bride." Everyone completed the toast. The newlyweds cut and distributed the top layer of cake.

Before the Governor and Ellen left to attend to an emergency in Denver, Jessica asked about the Chinese consulate in Denver. Her father explained, "I've met the new consul. Very polished with a hint of a British accent. I'm not sure they're open for business yet, because the virus has delayed everything. I'll check into it for you."

Marlene and Norma helped Roger put the cabin back to normal while Jessica changed into jeans. When the foursome sat down with real champagne, Norma asked, "Is there a honeymoon?"

Roger answered, "Jessica has agreed to go to Tibet for the trip I started before the accident."

"It's a fascinating adventure. I hope this pandemic gets done so we can travel again. I've already found an internet course on wildlife photography to get my skill closer to Roger's."

When the champagne bottle was empty, the two witnesses repeated their best wishes and said their goodbyes.

Jessica asked Roger, "Do you think everyone was shocked at the wedding feast?"

"Hell, no. They all know your penchant for pizza, and there was no opportunity for a banquet. The cake was great; what are we going to do with the bottom layer?" he asked.

"I'll wrap it well and freeze it. We can serve it at the celebration we promised everyone in Denver."

CHAPTER 28

The day after the wedding, the governor called Jessica. "The new Chinese consulate isn't open for business yet, but they are close. The consul, Xi Chen, suggests you fill out the visa and permit applications and send them to him for processing. He will get back to you about an appointment when the consulate is open. He warned that it could be some weeks." He gave her the consulate address.

Together at her desk, Roger and Jessica completed the forms from the internet, following the instructions of "ALL BLOCK LETTERS NO HANDWRITING OR CORRECTIONS ALLOWED." They posted a large envelope the next day.

After the wedding, they amended their routine. Jessica fielded one or two calls per day from the Governor's office. For the remainder of her day, she continued researching Tibet, practicing her photography skills, and expanding her culinary repertoire. Roger spent his mornings developing his plans for the institute. He resumed his communication with the two academic candidates, Lawrence Guttman at UC Berkely and Jocelyn Williams at UCSF. Both were completing post-doctoral programs after obtaining PhDs.

Guttman had already published two papers on his success in creating brainoids. He had drafted a grant application and was anxious to find a permanent academic home from which to apply. He was familiar with Denver, was an avid skier, and had a stellar academic record. His post-doctoral supervisor gave him a glowing recommendation and expressed regret that he could not offer him a job. Roger was aware Iowa and Michigan were also courting Guttman.

Roger renewed their previous email relationship and suggested they arrange a zoom or skype call. Guttman responded immediately, and they calendared a zoom call for the next morning. The call lasted two hours. The two men found much in common, especially concerning the need for more innovative implants, such as Guttman's brainoids. Roger convinced him that funding for equipment was almost certain, given the Institute's backing. Guttman did not question Roger's salary offer, which included moving expenses. That settled, Guttman had a suggestion. For the past two years, he had partially supervised a PhD candidate in their department. Hanson Fong, from Hong Kong, was due to defend his thesis later in the month. Assuming he was successful, Fong would then be seeking a post-doctoral position. Guttman asked Roger, "Is there any possibility of offering him a two-year post-doc with us?"

Although surprised at the request, Roger was delighted; he was hiring a team, not an individual. "I think we can do that, but I have to get approval from the dean and my funding source. Give me a week to work on it. Did you say you can start June 1, virus permitting?" When Guttman assented, Roger explained a formal appointment letter would follow within the week for Guttman's position as Assistant Professor. Now that Guttman was on board, Roger would work on the Williams candidate.

Over lunch, Roger shared the news with Jessica, who commented,

"I'm glad to see you're going back to work instead of moping about your identity and medical license."

"I have to believe we'll solve the identity issue, and I see that I'll have almost no opportunity for patient contact. The medical license doesn't mean that much to me. I still think of myself as a doctor. It's now been two weeks since we sent in the visa applications. How long will they take to reply?" Roger asked.

"The consul warned it would take a while. I'll wait another week before I try to follow up."

A week later, Jessica phoned the consulate and heard a recorded voice message suggesting that any caller should leave a message. Jessica said, "This is Jessica Lupen. Some weeks ago, my husband Roger Scully and I applied for visas and Tibet permits. We need to plan our travel, so we would appreciate a progress report."

Three days later, an envelope addressed to Jessica arrived from the Chinese consulate. With eager anticipation, Jessica tore it open. There was only one line of text: *The applications from you and Mr. Scully are not approved.* Xi Chen had signed the letter. Jessica gasped, "Look at this letter. No explanation, no reasons, and no mention of how we can appeal. What should we do?"

"Call your Dad. He knows the consul."

The governor suggested they ask for an appointment with the consul to seek an explanation. "I'll call ahead and tell them to expect you to ask for an appointment. They don't want to offend the governor, so you'll probably get to see Chen. I have no idea what he'll say to explain this."

The next day, a female consulate employee called Jessica to offer an appointment with the consul the following week. Jessica accepted and approached Roger at his folding-table desk. "We're on for next Tuesday afternoon. What do you think will happen?"

"I haven't a clue. It might have nothing to do with us. Perhaps the virus has all visa applications stopped. We'll see. Maybe we can use my Chinese citizenship as Wu Zicheng to get your visa. I won't need one."

"You'd do that? I thought you had given up your Chinese citizenship," Jessica said.

"No, I never gave it up. That guy took my passport in Hong Kong, but I'm still a Chinese citizen. I'll take some passport photos so the consul can renew my passport while we're there."

"I think you should call the consulate and warn them you will be there to get a new passport at the visit," Jessica advised.

"Good idea." When he telephoned the consulate he heard the same recorded message, so he left a voicemail explaining that Wu Zicheng would be applying for a new passport.

Jessica and Roger entered the consular offices with some enthusiasm and a hope they could solve the travel problems. A smiling receptionist said, "You are expected. Please come and meet Consul Chen." She ushered them into a small conference room. When they were seated, a tall and distinguished-looking man appeared and sat at the head of the table. He nodded at being introduced but made no attempt to shake hands.

His face was impassive. "What is the reason for your visit?" he asked.

Jessica spoke up, "You denied our visa applications. We want to know why and find out about an appeal mechanism."

Before Chen could answer, Roger added, "And I'd like to get a new passport for Wu Zucheng."

"The central authority denied the visas. I have no knowledge of their reasons. There is no appeal mechanism."

Jessica and Roger looked disappointed, but Roger pressed on, "And my new passport?"

"Our records have no evidence that Wu Zicheng ever existed," Chen said, still with no change of facial expression.

Roger stood up with an angry expression. "What is this bullshit? You know my story about the transplant. How can you sit there and deny my history?"

"My instructions and information come from higher authorities. I remind you that this appointment is highly irregular. I granted it only as a favor to Governor Lupen. Your business here is finished. Good day." He rose and left the room after pressing a button.

The receptionist re-entered the room. With a slight smile, she said, "Let me show you out."

Jessica drove them back to Loveland; Roger was too distraught. After a string of curses, he said, "The bastards have taken away my being. A few weeks ago, I had two identities; now I have none."

"I'm very disappointed. When Dad managed to get our appointment, I was sure it would all work out. It's not just the loss of our honeymoon trip. It's what they've done to you," Jessica said.

"I need to think about this," Roger said, lapsing into silence with his head on his chest.

On arrival at the Loveland Cabin, Roger headed for his laptop, where his fingers started flying over the keys. With a puzzled look, Jessica stood behind him, reading the words as they appeared.

Dear Mr. Moon:

I am writing to you out of desperation…

He continued with a lengthy explanation of his life since his return to the US, his loss of medical license, his academic position, and his recent marriage and honeymoon plans. He mentioned he would be receiving a Chinese post-doctoral student within a few months. In his final paragraph, he wrote:

Your foresight and support of the Harbin team not only saved my life, you changed the lives of dozens of other people who now benefit from the surgical discoveries at Harbin. I don't know if you can help me, but I want to re-establish my identity as Wu Ziteng and take my bride to China and Tibet.

Thank you for all you have done for me. I owe you my life.

Sincerely, Wu Ziteng.

"Wow, that's quite a letter. Do you think it'll work?" asked Jessica.

"I haven't a clue, but I can't think of anything else."

Three days later, the consular receptionist called and asked to speak to Wu Ziteng. In a cool and detached voice, she said, "Doctor Wu, if you and your wife present yourself at the consulate tomorrow morning with sets of appropriate pictures, your new passport and your wife's six-month travel visa can be issued the same day."

Jessica was listening on the speakerphone, her arms on Roger's shoulders as he sat. He leaped upright and shouted, "Fucking-A, it worked. Let's do the trip!" as he hugged Jessica.

On September 2, Wu Ziteng and Jessica Lupen met their guide at the Lhas Gonggar airport in Tibet. According to all available records, Roger Scully is still dead. On the same day, in Shenzen, Zhao Lushan filed a birth certificate for her newborn son, Zhao Ziteng. She did not identify the father on the document.

Epilogue

Since finishing the novel, the Chinese government has published a price list of organs for transplant. Children's parts have a different price list. Brains are not yet listed as available. Every day in the United States, seventeen people die awaiting transplants. Our society should do better. I am not advocating the Chinese solution, but prisoners should be able to donate unpaired organs or liver lobes in return for money and/or sentence reduction.

For readers with a continuing interest in Dr. Scully, I will be setting up a webpage to invite solutions as to how he might regain his identity and medical license. I look forward to your responses.

Acknowledgements

Bonnie Shelton, my first editor, pushed me through my first attempt at fiction to make this novel. Miciah Bay Gault mentored me through the Vermont School of Fine Arts summer program. Holly Coale and Marina Muldowney provided encouragement, criticism and hours of reading aloud. My final editor, Kevin Breen, supplied reams of critical comments to finish the work. The polished finished product reflects the artistry of David Prendergast. To all I say, thank you. I could not have done it alone.